D0453830

"Butler and Lewis have updated t[...] and useful work, covering with thoroughness all physical and psychological aspects of sex and romance after six decades of life. The skill with which they clear away the clutter of prejudice and show that dysfunction is a result of Something Wrong (often quite correctable) and not a matter of age, makes great reading." —Hugh Downs

"Every man and woman over 60 needs Dr. Butler to be their personal physician and counselor, and since that's not possible, this book, full of information and reassurance, is the next best thing." —Eda LeShan

"Love & Sex After 60 emphasizes the importance of love and sex as integral components of human interactions in all phases in life, even as men and women age. This important contribution will be enthusiastically received."
—Michael J. Droller, M.D., Professor and Chairman, Department of Urology, The Mount Sinai Medical Center, and Chair of the Consensus Conference on Impotence at the National Institutes of Health

"This extraordinary book fills an information vacuum for men and women over 60, an ever expanding segment of our population. Every man and woman needs this book, for if they are not now over sixty, hopefully someday they will be."
—E. Douglas Whitehead, M.D., F.A.C.S.

"A wonderful affirmation that sexuality is a natural and healthy part of living throughout our lives. A great 60th birthday present." —Debra W. Haffner, M.P.H., Executive Director, Sex Information and Education Council of the United States

LOVE AND SEX

AFTER 60

REVISED EDITION

ROBERT N. BUTLER, M.D.

AND MYRNA I. LEWIS, M.S.W.

A LONG LIFE BOOK

BALLANTINE BOOKS · NEW YORK

CONTENTS

CONTENTS

PREFACE

How times have changed! When we wrote the first edition of *Love and Sex After 60* in 1976, the subject made many people uncomfortable—in fact, it was almost a taboo topic. In a move typical of this skittish attitude, a Florida newspaper refused to advertise the book's publication, saying it was too prurient for the public. When we were appearing on network television, the interviewer warned parents to keep their teenagers and small children out of the room, away from the "dangerous" topic of late-life sexuality. (And yet now families are watching Geraldo, Donohue, and Oprah!) Health professionals admitted that they rarely, if ever, discussed sexuality as part of their medical and psychological evaluation of older people. The media treated the subject with ridicule and disparagement—if they addressed it at all. And many older people themselves were unclear about the propriety of sexuality at that point in their lives.

In the face of all this negativity, how did we become involved in writing about love and sex after sixty? Well, for years a number of older people had come to see us in our psychotherapy practices, insisting that their sexuality be taken seriously. They wanted advice on how to maintain relationships, whether old or new. They wanted help with physical problems that were interfering with their sexuality. They wanted their families, their doctors, and the world in general to recognize them as full, functioning adults. It dawned on us that they needed a book of their own on the vital topic of late-life sexuality.

Nearly twenty years have passed since then. The subject is no longer taboo. The sexuality of older people has become a generally accepted fact of life. Even TV sitcoms portray older persons conducting romances and maintaining relationships that clearly involve sexuality. But easy access to reliable and up-to-date information on late-life sexuality still remains problematic for many. Moreover, a surprising number of older people want the chance to learn how to keep relationships that have either lasted a long time or are being created anew alive and fulfilling in their later years. These demands have led us to the task of revising the material in this book.

Our aim in this newest edition is to continue to

bring older people the latest information on the dynamic subject of sexuality. There is much that is new and heartening, but there are still negative stereotypes to challenge. And there is much that is continuing to evolve in the understanding of the physical and psychological issues of late-life sexuality. The diagnosis and treatment of sexual problems *have* greatly improved. Health professionals, the public, and older people themselves have become more aware of the continuing importance of sexuality as one grows older. And we humans seem to be gradually maturing in our capacity to recognize that the added gift of life—an average of twenty-five more years of life expectancy since the turn of the century—is giving us an unprecedented opportunity to develop the art of living and loving more richly and fully.

ACKNOWLEDGMENTS

We would like to acknowledge the following people for their much-appreciated help with this revision: Mia Oberlink and Fergal O'Doherty for their research and editing; Dr. E. Douglas Whitehead, urologist, for his technical review of erectile dysfunction treatments; and Dr. Diane Meier, a geriatrician and internist, for reviewing the material on osteoporosis. We are especially grateful to our editor, Elizabeth Zack, at Ballantine Books.

LOVE AND SEX
AFTER 60

CHAPTER 1

LOVE AND SEX AFTER SIXTY

Frank and Marietta have been married forty-six years. At first glance, their lives have not been especially remarkable, and in fact, they have had their share of tragedies. Yet these two positively glow with humor and enthusiasm. Frank says of Marietta, "I love this woman more each day." And Marietta answers, "I couldn't have asked for a better partner—kind, sweet, sexy, and funny. He is everything a woman could want." Both are quick to declare that it is their relationship that has been the core of their sense of satisfaction in life.

Our society is in the midst of a longevity revolution. We have gained twenty-eight years of average life expectancy in the past ninety some years. Every day 6,000

Americans turn sixty. Altogether, forty-two million people, or one out of every six of us, is sixty or older. What happens to our sexuality at this time of life? Many people—not only the young and middle-aged but older people themselves—simply assume that it is over. They couldn't be more wrong. Our own clinical and research work, the work of other gerontologists, the research of Kinsey, and the clinical discoveries of Masters and Johnson all demonstrate that relatively healthy older people who enjoy sex are capable of experiencing it—often until *very* late in life. Frequently those who do have sexual problems can be helped.

We have written this book for those older men and women who are presently or potentially interested in sexuality and would like to know more about what is likely to happen to their sexuality over time. We will offer solutions to sexual problems that may occur, and propose ways of countering the negative attitudes that older people may experience—within themselves, from family members, from the medical and psychotherapeutic professions, and from society at large. We especially want older people to know that their concerns and problems are not unique, that they are not alone in their experience, and that many others feel *exactly as they do*. Even those people who have had a lively enthusiasm and capacity for sex all their lives often need information, support, and sometimes various kinds of treatment in order to continue engaging in sexual activity as the years go by. In addition, people for whom sex may not have been especially satisfying in their younger days may find that it is now possible to improve the quality of the experience despite their long-standing difficulties.

Sex and sexuality are pleasurable, rewarding, and fulfilling experiences that can enhance the later years. But they are also—as everyone knows—enormously complex psychologically. Every one of us carries with us throughout our lives a weight of infant and childhood experiences related to sex that have been shaped by ourselves, our parents, our families, our teachers, and our society, some of which are positive and some negative, some of which we realize and many of which we are unaware.

Because of this, it is useful to understand what underlies so many of the attitudes and problems about sex that one encounters. If you are an older person, be prepared for the likelihood of conflicting feelings within yourself and contradictory attitudes from the outside world. Should older people have sex lives? Are they even able to make love? Do they really want to? Is it appropriate—that is, "normal" or "decent"—or is sexual interest a sign of "senility" and brain disease (he/she has gone "daft"), poor judgment, or an embarrassing inability to adjust to aging with the proper restraint and resignation?

How much less troubling it would be to accept the folklore of cookie-baking grandmothers who bustle about the kitchen making goodies for their loved ones while rocking-chair grandfathers puff on their pipes and

reminisce. Idealized folk figures like these are not supposed to have sex lives of their own. After all, they are
our parents and grandparents, not ordinary adults with
the same needs and desires that we have.

As an older man or woman, you may find that love
and sex in later life, when they are acknowledged at all,
will be patronizingly thought of as "cute" or "sweet,"
like the puppy love of teenagers; but even more likely,
they will be ridiculed, a subject for jokes that have un-
dercurrents of disdain and apprehensiveness at the pros-
pect of growing older. Our language is full of telltale
phrases: older men become "dirty old men," "old
fools," or "old goats" where sex is involved. Older
women are often depicted as "old hags." Most of this
"humor" implies the impotence of older men and the
ugliness of older women.

A mythology fed by misinformation surrounds late-
life sexuality. The presumption is that sexual desire automatically ebbs with age—that it begins to decline
when you are in your forties, proceeds relentlessly
downward (you are "losing it"), and eventually hits bot-
tom (you are "over the hill") at some time between sixty
and sixty-five. Thus an older woman who shows an
evident, perhaps even a lusty, interest in sex is often
assumed to be suffering from "emotional" problems;
and if she is obviously in her right mind and sexually
active, she runs the risk of being called "depraved" or,
more kindly, said to be clinging pathetically to her lost
youth.

Lustiness in young men is often seen as lechery in older men, a sign of inappropriate emotional lapse. Therefore older men may find themselves the objects of sexual suspicion. Even simple affection can be misunderstood. An older man's show of warmth toward children other than his own grandchildren or those of his friends runs the risk of an assumption that it is sexually tinged. How real is this danger? According to crime statistics, child molesting, popularly associated with older men, is actually committed primarily by young men in their twenties.

From time to time everybody is caught up by accounts of older people who perform sexual feats "despite" their age. Newspapers relish them: "92-year-old-man is father of twins"; "Woman of 73 and man of 76 arrested by police in love nest"; "Judge of 81 marries 22-year-old showgirl"; "72-year-old woman jailed for attempted prostitution." In the popular mind these older people walk the thin line between sexual heroics and indecency, with part of the public saying "More power to them" and the remainder reacting with disgust. Everyone, however, reads the accounts with the mixture of revulsion and fascination reserved for the extraordinary and the bizarre.

Why are we still so negative about sex in later life and about older people in general? Much of this attitude is an outgrowth of our own fear of growing old and dying, and it has given rise to a prejudice we have called *ageism*, which is a systematic discrimination against people because they are old, just as racism and sexism discriminate for reasons of skin color and gender. The ageist sees older people in stereotypes: rigid, boringly talkative, senile, old-fashioned in morality and lacking in skills, useless, and with little redeeming social value. There's a fine irony in the fact that if the ageists live long enough they are going to end up being "old" themselves and the victims, in turn, of their own prejudice; their attitude will culminate in self-hatred. A great many older people have fallen into this trap, often at devastating cost to their personal happiness. And as far as sexuality is concerned, ageism says if you are getting old, you're finished.

Some of these attitudes are rooted in our relatively recent past. At the turn of the century, when the average life expectancy was forty-seven years, few older people lived to old age and fewer still were healthy enough to be sexually active. But today life expectancy is seventy-five years and we have a large population of relatively healthy people over sixty-five. Of these, 95 percent live in the community, 81 percent can get around by themselves, and about 30 percent are still working part- or full-time. (We now term the age period sixty-five to seventy-four "early old age" and call that over seventy-five "later old age.") Yet we have not accepted these new realities, nor have popular attitudes caught up; the general image of late life still assumes frailty or decrepitude as par for the course.

If we join these cultural attitudes with the prevalent

sexual "yardsticks" by which we are all influenced, it is no wonder that older people may be confused and uncertain about sex! Both men and women worry about "wearing out" physically. They want to know what changes are to be expected with normal aging, whether there is reasonable hope for a physically healthy and active sex life, and whether lovemaking can be as good as it was when they were younger.

Men especially are victims of a lifelong excessive emphasis on physical performance. Masculinity is equated with physical prowess. Older men judge themselves and are judged by comparing the frequency and potency of their sexual performance with that of younger men. But these comparisons seldom place any value on experience and on the quality of the sex. When measured by standards that are essentially athletic, older men naturally are considered inferior. And so they often panic at the first sign of change: "Lately I've been troubled by the fact that I seem to take longer to have a good erection. Is something wrong? Am I becoming impotent? Will I be able to have a firm erection as I get older? Will sex be as pleasurable as when I was younger? Will my partner think I am inadequate?"

In terms of performance, women are under less pressure, of course, but they, too, worry about changes. They may report they are losing their "grip"—namely the muscle strength in the vagina that enables them to hold a penis. The size of the vagina itself may change, and there may be problems with "dryness" as vaginal lubrication lessens. Some women begin to experience pain during intercourse and want to know what to do to eliminate it.

But the predominant pressure on women comes from what can be termed "aesthetic narrowness," that widespread assumption that only the young are beautiful. Many older people believe this themselves. When a woman's hair turns gray and her skin develops wrinkles and her body loses its earlier firmness and suppleness, she is very likely to see herself as unattractive. The idea of beauty desperately needs to be revised to include character, intelligence, expressiveness, knowledge, achievement, disposition, tone of voice and speech patterns, posture and bearing, warmth, personal style, social skills—all those personal traits that make each individual unique and that can be found at *any* age.

In late life we find just as many complaints between partners about sexual incompatibilities as at any other time: interest on one side and disinterest on the other, or passivity, or rebuffs, or failure to agree on the frequency of lovemaking. We get comments like the following all the time:

I am in good health at age sixty-five and so is my sixty-three-year-old wife. She is a wonderful person, and she did a beautiful job rearing five children. The problem—sex. On my sixty-third birthday she did me the grand "favor" of sleeping with me. She then announced that from now on I'd better forget about sex because, as she put it, "We are too old to carry on like this." I don't feel old. I am still full of energy.

Problems also arise between couples when one partner is incapacitated or chronically ill and the other is healthy. If the healthy partner has active sexual needs, anger and irritation at being denied the opportunity to express sexuality often lead to guilt, as if one were lacking the appropriate concern and compassion for the ailing partner. The latter, in turn, may feel guilty at being unable to participate fully in lovemaking.

Tension in the later years often arises when those who are parents are inhibited by their sons and daughters, who find it uncomfortable to accept sexuality in their mothers and fathers. (We all agree that *our* parents were *never* interested in sex!) Many adults continue to be bound by a primitive childhood need to deny their parents a sex life and to lock them into purely parental roles. For these children their parents are never fellow adults. Nor are their motivations always psychological. Avarice and selfishness, unhappily enough, are common. If one parent dies, children may deliberately try to prevent the surviving parent from meeting new friends (and potential new partners) in order to protect their inheritance. Any evidence of parental sexuality or romance threatens them and their inheritance.

And what of the older lesbian and gay population,

perhaps one out of every ten of us? We have included a brief section on lesbian and gay relationships on page 221. We hope it is an important beginning in encouraging dialogue and research on the specific concerns of elderly lesbians and gays.

We have now sketched out a number of ways—both positive and negative—in which individuals and society react to sex in older people. But what about those of you who are not particularly interested in sex? Many older people do feel this way. We want to emphasize that sexual disinterest is a matter of concern *only* if you find it personally troubling or if it causes problems in relating to others. Some people were never significantly interested in sex even when younger, whether because of their biological makeup or, more often, as a result of social conditioning. For others sex represents emotional conflict resulting from or causing difficult relations with their partners. For them and their partners the opportunity to discontinue sex under the socially acceptable guise of "sexless old age" can be a great relief.

Others have simply grown tired of sex: "How well I remember the aged poet Sophocles' response to the question 'How does love sit with age, Sophocles: are you still the man you were?' 'Peace,' he replied. 'Most gladly have I escaped that of which you speak: I feel as if I had escaped from a mad and furious monster.' "* If sex had

*From the *Dialogues of Plato*, 4th ed. New York: Clarendon Press, 1953, p. 165.

been shared with the same partner routinely for years, many may now have compensated for its dullness by developing satisfying nonsexual activities. Other people may have stopped having sex because of disabilities or serious illnesses. When their health improved there may have been no motivation to change what had become a comfortable habit. Sometimes an individual will have made a deliberate decision to share sex only with a particular partner, and thus, when illness or death intervened, his or her experience of sex came to a close. Other people view sex as only for the purpose of procreation, not for pleasure, and feel their religion supports this conviction, so sex ends with the completion of menopause. Self-imposed abstinence from sex may also be simply the continuation of a lifelong habit. This can often be traced back to frightening early experiences or to feelings that sex is forbidden and dangerous, and the avoidance of sex altogether may provide an adjustment that works reasonably well.

Whatever the reasons, it *is* possible to live a happy and satisfying life without sex if that is one's choice, and a good many older people do exactly that. The American emphasis on sexuality has had the effect of making many of the young and middle-aged feel guilty, inadequate, or incomplete if sex fails to play a central role in their lives; we do not want to place a similar burden on older people. Those who have neither a desire for nor an interest in sex, or who have deliberately chosen a lifestyle in which sexuality plays little or no part, *are* entitled to live the life they find most fulfilling.

On the other hand, those older people who do enjoy sex *deserve* encouragement and support, as well as necessary information and appropriate treatment if problems arise. Sexuality—the physical and emotional responsiveness to sexual stimuli—goes beyond the sex urge and the sex act. For many older people it offers the opportunity to express not only passion but affection, esteem, and loyalty. It provides affirmative evidence that one can count on one's body and its functioning. It allows people to assert themselves positively. It carries with it the possibility of excitement and romance; it expresses delight in being alive. It offers a continuous challenge to grow and change in new directions.

CHAPTER 2

❧～❧

NORMAL PHYSICAL CHANGES IN SEXUALITY THAT OCCUR WITH AGE

What happens to your body sexually as it ages? While there are significant changes in the physical and physiological aspects of sex as you age, in the absence of disease or adverse drug effects, such changes do not usually cause sexual problems.

The act of sex is complex, for it encompasses the body, the mind, and the emotions. It involves the nervous system and the hormones as well as specific organs of the body. All of these participate in the sexual-response cycle, which includes sexual desire, followed by excitement or erotic arousal, orgasm or climax, and resolution or recovery. Both men and women experience similar sexual responses.

People are stimulated sexually in a number of

ways—through sight, smell, touch, thoughts, and feelings. The pelvic area reacts. Muscle tension and congestion (filling of the blood vessels) occur, especially in the sexual or genital organs. The sex hormones that play an active role in this responsiveness are steroids, produced in the adrenal glands of both men and women and in the ovaries of women and the testes of men. Estrogen, one of the active female hormones, has a profound effect on the development and functioning of the female sex organs. Androgen, the primary male hormone, appears to influence sexual desire in both men and women (women have small amounts of androgen) as well as sexual development and performance in men. It's the body's master gland, the pituitary, which is located in the brain, that affects the levels of all hormones, including the sex hormones. And as men and women age, the changes in their bodies affect their sexuality in different ways.

OLDER WOMEN

Most of the sexual changes in women can be directly traced to the decline of female hormones, especially estrogen, associated with menopause. Menopause, also called the "change of life" or "climacteric," is a physiological process that continues for several years and takes place anywhere between the ages of forty-five and fifty-five, with an average age of fifty to fifty-two. It involves fluctuations in estrogen levels from previously normal levels (prior to menopause) to near zero. Its most conspicuous sign is the cessation of menstruation.

Although 85 percent of women experience hot flashes and other menopausal symptoms during menopause, only about 20 percent actually seek medical attention. It appears that many simply are not bothered enough by their symptoms to look for medical help; others are not aware of current medical interventions or cannot afford them. It is estimated that perhaps 25 percent of all women, at the time of their menopause, will have symptoms that, if left untreated, interfere in some important way with their lives. Somewhat later, larger numbers of women will experience thinning of the vaginal walls as well as what is called "stress," or "urge," incontinence (see page 70). Much later, many will develop the brittle bones and the tendency toward back pain and fractures that are typical of advanced osteoporosis, a condition exacerbated by the loss of estrogen in the postmenopausal years. Atherosclerosis in women in later life is also thought to be accelerated by the estrogen loss. (Both osteoporosis and atherosclerosis in relation to estrogen will be discussed later in this chapter.) The following are examples of how differently menopause can affect individual women and their life-styles.

Once her menopause began, Greta could hardly sleep at night. She would wake up drenched in sweat, totally alert, with her adrenaline flowing. It would be difficult to get to sleep again. When she did fall asleep again, she would awaken shortly thereafter in another devastating sweat that would leave her exhausted. After her sleep loss began to accumulate, she became irritable and depressed. She and her husband began to argue with each other. Greta grew more and more disconsolate and eventually went to her physician in despair, thinking she was losing her mind. Her internist tried tranquilizers. But eventually Greta saw her gynecologist, who prescribed short-term estrogen replacement therapy, which helped significantly. Her hot flashes, night sweats, irritability, and fatigue quickly disappeared. She and her gynecologist are now trying to decide whether long-term estrogen/progestin is indicated.

Florence, on the other hand, went through her menopause without apparent symptoms, as do about 15 percent of all women. In fact, the onset of menopause made her feel somewhat liberated. She and her husband had long since decided that three children were enough. Despite her use of contraception, she had always had a nagging concern that she might have an unwanted midlife pregnancy. Her husband, Philip, was delighted for her and for himself when they no longer had this concern and were free of the need to use birth control. Thus menopause affects women and their partners in vastly different ways.

Common symptoms resulting from the hormonal imbalance menopause causes may include hot flashes, headaches and neckaches, excessive fatigue, and feelings of emotional instability. Yet, none of these are inevitable, and when they do occur, they can often be greatly alleviated or sometimes relieved entirely by various treatments. Life stresses can also precipitate or exacerbate these menopausal symptoms, and under those circumstances psychological counseling can be helpful. But even when left untreated, certain menopausal symptoms, like hot flashes, can subside spontaneously in time.

During or, more usually, following menopause, large numbers of older women begin to show signs of estrogen or sex-steroid deprivation, which can affect their sexual functioning. Elizabeth, sixty-five, had experienced pain during intercourse in the first ten years after her menopause, which took place when she was fifty-one. She and her husband had given up making love once she turned sixty-one, much to her relief: The pain had not been worth the pleasure. When we saw her, we learned that her doctor had never inquired about any sexual problems, and that she in turn had been too embarrassed to discuss her vaginal pain and occasional vaginal bleeding. We quickly referred her for an evaluation and treatment. In her case, it simply meant using vaginal lubricants that could be purchased over the counter at her local pharmacy. Elizabeth and her husband began experimenting, tentatively at first, with resuming their sexual relationship. To her delight, Elizabeth discovered that she was pain-free.

Many women, like Elizabeth, do complain of a feeling of "dryness" or "loss of juices" in the vagina, particularly during sexual intercourse. (Vaginal lubrication produced by congestion of the blood vessels in the vaginal wall is the physiological equivalent of erection in the man.) Lubrication of the walls of the vagina begins to take longer as a woman grows older. This seems to be due both to the loss of the estrogen necessary to produce appropriate secretions and to changes in the structure of the vaginal wall itself, through which the secretions ooze. When this happens, intercourse may feel scratchy, rough, and eventually painful.

Typically, the lining of the vagina begins to thin and become easily irritated, leading to pain and sometimes to cracking and bleeding both during and after intercourse. The vagina is less able to absorb the shock of a thrusting penis. Such pain (dyspareunia) occurs especially if the intercourse is of a long duration or if it follows a long period without sexual contact. Sometimes the shape of the vagina itself changes, becoming narrower, shorter, and less elastic, although generally it continues to be more than large enough for intercourse. Hormone replacement therapy has often been effective for protection against vaginal atrophy and dryness. (See pages 26–33 for a more detailed discussion of this therapy.) Vaginal lubricants are also extremely useful in decreasing any pain.

Pain and discomfort of *any* kind in the vaginal area should always be taken seriously by women and their physicians since it obviously interferes with sexual pleasure and response. In many cases, but not always, physicians can tell during a vaginal exam whether a woman has vaginal atrophy severe enough to cause pain. Other causes of pain are vaginal dryness, endometriosis, a fixed retroverted uterus, a prolapsed ovary, or water in the Fallopian tubes (hydrosalpinx)—all of which need medical attention.

With the loss of estrogen the usually acid vaginal secretions become less acidic, increasing the possibility of vaginal infection and causing burning, itching, and discharge. This condition is variously called estrogen-deficient, steroid-deficient, atrophic, or "senile" vaginitis. It *is* curable, and should be treated by a doctor. Home douching should not be attempted unless your doctor instructs you to do so for some specific medical purpose; it can confuse the diagnosis and may not, in any case, be an effective treatment.

Do not assume, however, that all vaginal itching and discharge reflect an estrogen deficiency. There should be a complete examination, including a Pap test, to rule out the possibility of a tumor of the reproductive tract. Allergies, trichomoniasis, and yeast and fungus infections (especially in diabetics) are other causes of itching; womb prolapse (fallen womb) may produce a vaginal discharge.

With the thinning of the vaginal walls, the bladder and urethra (the tube through which the urine is passed) are less protected and may be irritated during intercourse. Older women can develop what is sometimes called "honeymoon cystitis," an inflammation of the bladder resulting from bruising and jostling, or from exposure to semen and bacteria in the sensitive vaginal area after a period of sexual abstinence.

Dorothy's inflammation of the bladder resulted from a weekend of sexual activity with her husband, which came after several years of abstinence. Her husband had had a heart attack two years before and had been fearful about engaging in sexual activity. Dorothy herself had been even more worried than him about the possible harmful effects. But now their doctor had reassured them that they could safely resume sex. What he forgot to warn them of was the possibility of honeymoon cystitis, a kind of disuse problem. Fortunately, the situation quickly resolved itself; Dorothy's vaginal tract soon adjusted to the presence of bacterial substances resulting from intercourse.

Honeymoon cystitis at first is simply irritating, but when bacteria are present, it can become a full-fledged cystitis, characterized by an unrelenting, irresistible urge to urinate and accompanied by a burning sensation. This condition must be treated medically. Advanced stages bring an increasingly painful burning during urination, waking at night to urinate, and, occasionally, blood in the urine. Such infections require prompt medical attention when they occur.

As women age they might also notice that the clitoris may slightly reduce in size (although this is not always the case). The lips of the vagina (the labia) may become less firm. The covering of the clitoris and the fat pad in the hair-covered pubic area lose some of their fatty tissue, leaving the clitoris less protected and more easily irritated. However, be aware that clitoral stimulation continues to be a source of intense sexual sensation and orgasm, essentially as it was in earlier years.

Women in good health who were able to have orgasms in their younger years can continue having orgasms until very late in life—until well into their eighties or even later. Indeed, some women begin to have orgasms for the first time as they grow older. The lack of orgasmic ability earlier in life does not necessarily mean that such a pattern will continue if a woman eventually learns how to understand and manage her own sexual response. What is unclear, however, is whether the length of time required to reach orgasm changes as women age. Nor do we know for certain whether age affects the duration and intensity of an orgasm. Shorter-lasting orgasms and spasms in the uterus, when they occur, may be evidence of a hormonal imbalance.

So, except for the effects of estrogen loss after menopause, the normal physical changes that accompany aging interfere very little with a female's sexual ability. Reports of a decline in women's sexual interest as they age seem to be predominantly psychologically defensive or protective in origin rather than physiological. The actual frequency of sexual intercourse in women tends to be more affected by their partners' age, health, and level of sexual interest and functioning than a reflection of reduced interest or capacity in women themselves.

Older women are the best witnesses on this issue of continuing sexual interest. Here is a letter we received from a seventy-two-year-old woman:

It's about time that someone acknowledged and brought out of the closet the subject of sexual desire and activity for those of us in our later years. I live in a senior citizens' apartment building where 95 percent of the tenants are women. There are four or five widowers here, but none of them are currently being pursued by a woman. Isn't this pathetic? People here are too sedentary. Unfortunately, none of these men are personally appealing to me or I would take action. . . . At my age I still consider myself attractive enough for any man, maybe even one a few years younger than myself. All I need to know now is "Where the Boys Are."

Our reply.

Thank you for your wonderful letter. It is great to hear from readers as lively and enthusiastic as you. We share your concerns about "where the boys are." As you know, there is no easy answer to this question. Men will sooner or later have to learn to live healthier lives so they don't die off so quickly! In the meantime, it is a delight to hear from someone as spirited as you, even when an interesting man is not available.

TREATMENT OF POSTMENOPAUSAL CHANGES

Regular Sexual Activity

Although still controversial, there is some evidence that regular sexual activity helps preserve functioning, especially lubricatory ability, and may even stimulate estrogen production. Sexually active women also seem to have less vaginal atrophy. The regular muscle contractions during sexual activity and orgasm do maintain vaginal muscle tone, and it is thought that intercourse helps preserve the shape and size of the vaginal space.

Yet following the death or illness of a partner, many women find themselves without the opportunity for sexual contact. If it is psychologically acceptable, self-stimulation (masturbation) can be effective in preserving lubricating ability and the muscle tone that maintains the size and shape of the vagina. In addition, it can release tension, stimulate sexual appetite, and contribute to general well-being. Self-stimulation is probably more common among younger women because they have grown up in a less restrictive sexual atmosphere. But it seems clear that it is being practiced by women of all ages with growing frequency, lessened anxiety, and considerable physical benefit. In fact, masturbation is increasingly viewed not only as a response to the loss of sexual contact with a partner but also as a natural and ongoing supplementary activity within a relationship.

Hormone Replacement Therapy

The popularity of estrogen replacement therapy (ERT) has had its ups and downs in recent years. Estrogen was first used to treat the problems of menopause in the late 1940s. The use of estrogen in its most popular form, Premarin, gained momentum throughout the 1960s and the mid-1970s, fueled by physician Robert Wilson's popular book, *Feminine Forever*. Estrogen replacement therapy was promoted as a protection against hot flashes, backache, memory loss, vaginal atrophy, depression, lowered sex drive, and such general aging signs as wrinkles and gray hair. Common side effects were thought to be occasional dose-related uterine bleeding and minor complaints of nausea, fluid retention, weight gain, and increased susceptibility to vaginal yeast infection. By 1975, about 6 million women were receiving ERT.

However, ERT usage declined sharply after five studies in 1975–76 showed it was associated with an increased risk of endometrial cancer (cancer affecting the lining of the uterus)—especially if ERT had been given for more than five years. Both women and their physicians became wary. But after several more years, researchers learned that adding progestin (a synthetic form of the female hormone progesterone) counters, and perhaps avoids altogether, the buildup in the endometrium that leads to endometrial cancer. With this news, the use of hormone replacement therapy (HRT), this time combining estrogen—in lower doses than formerly—and progestin, began to climb again. By 1990, more than 16 million American women were receiving some form of HRT.

Newer developments have brought added promise, as well as controversy and challenge, to the question of HRT use. Recent studies, including the ongoing Boston-based Nurses' Health Study of 48,470 postmenopausal women with no previous heart disease, have supported earlier observations that estrogen has preventive and life-lengthening effects against both heart disease and osteoporosis. This has catapulted hormone replacement therapy into use as a treatment for conditions other than menopause. Growing numbers of women over fifty are now reassessing estrogen use as a possible lifelong protection against heart disease, the greatest cause of death among women, and osteoporosis, one of the major causes of female disability in later life. Yet what is still worrisome is a possible link between estrogen and the development of breast cancer. Further, we currently know little about the long-term effects of adding progestin to the hormone replacement regimen, for it may possibly interfere with estrogen's protection against heart disease.

The biology of the menopause, which is still poorly understood, and these unresolved questions regarding postmenopausal hormone replacement therapy are now receiving increased attention at the National Institutes of Health (specifically the Postmenopausal Estrogen/ Progestin Interventions Trial, or PEPI study, at the National Heart, Lung and Blood Institute, as well as the Women's Health Initiative studies) and elsewhere. It is to be hoped that more information will soon be available for women and their physicians. The growing longevity of American women makes it *imperative* that the issues surrounding HRT use are clarified. Altogether, some 40 million American women are now postmenopausal, and as the baby-boom generation of women ages, nearly 70 million women will be postmenopausal by the year 2000.

BENEFITS OF HRT

The known risks and benefits of HRT must be evaluated individually by each woman and her physician. Hormone replacement therapy has short-term benefits for women with troublesome symptoms directly related to menopause. And in view of recent studies already mentioned, it appears that there also may be broader long-term health benefits as well:

Treatment of Menopausal Symptoms

Estrogen replacement is very effective in alleviating and, in most cases, eliminating many of the more immediate symptoms of menopause, especially hot flashes ("night sweats"), vaginal dryness, and thinning of the vaginal walls. And when hot flashes disappear, insomnia, irritability, and depression resulting from lack of sleep often improve dramatically. Some women also report fewer headaches and memory problems than they had during the menopausal period. Without added estrogen, many women begin to experience pain, discomfort, and even bleeding during intercourse.

Protection Against Heart Disease

Estrogen has been found to increase high density lipoproteins (HDLs—the "good" cholesterol) and decrease low density lipoproteins (LDLs—the dangerous cholesterol), which promote heart disease. It may also prevent the formation of fatty deposits in the arteries, which interfere with blood flow and can lead to both heart attacks and strokes. Women who do not take estrogen replacement risk a rapidly escalating incidence of heart disease after age sixty. In fact, heart disease is the leading cause of death in postmenopausal women.

Protection Against Osteoporosis

Estrogen slows the rapid bone loss that occurs during menopause and helps to prevent the thinning of the bones that leads to osteoporosis. This demineralizing disease affects 60 million postmenopausal women. It is the cause of bone fractures in 40 percent of women over seventy and can lead to broken hips, permanent disability, and death in many older women.

RISKS AND PROBLEMS
ASSOCIATED WITH HRT
Estrogen Risks

There is evidence that estrogen replacement can accelerate the development of preexisting estrogen-dependent cancers and of noncancerous fibroid tumors in the uterus. There is currently no clear evidence, however, that estrogen encourages the growth of new cancers, especially when a woman has been using estrogen for less than five years. Estrogen may also increase the risk of gallbladder disease, blood clots, hypertension, and PMS-like symptoms.

Who should *not* use estrogen? If you have any of the following conditions, your doctor will probably advise you to avoid taking estrogen:

• A known or suspected breast or uterine cancer or any other tumor that is stimulated by estrogen. Some physicians take the position that fibrocystic breast changes, fibroid tumors of the uterus, and endometriosis are also contraindications to taking estrogen.

• A strong family history of estrogen-dependent cancers.

- Diabetes.
- Blood clots of any kind, including thrombophlebitis, embolism, stroke, or heart attack.
- Chronic or acute liver disease.
- Abnormal or unexplained genital bleeding.
- Allergic reaction to estrogen.

Your doctor should also be cautious if you have high levels of fat or cholesterol in the blood, severe varicose veins, or very high blood pressure.

Progestin Problems

When progestin is added to the hormone replacement regimen as a protection against uterine cancer, some women experience side effects such as weight gain, abdominal bleeding, headaches, irritability, and breast tenderness. Others strongly object to the menstrual bleeding that occurs when progestin is taken on a cyclic schedule a certain number of days each month. (This bleeding is usually eliminated after the first few months if progestin is given on a continuous, low-dosage basis.) There is also evidence that progestin, especially when given in larger doses, interferes with the protective effect estrogen provides against heart disease.

Remember that not all women on hormone replacement therapy take progestin. For example, those who have had hysterectomies do not need progestin, since they have no uteruses. Other women, for a variety of reasons, choose to use estrogen alone, without progestin. It is strongly urged that such women have semiannual or at least yearly endometrial biopsies (a simple procedure that can be done in your doctor's office). Such biopsies can detect endometrial cancer in its early stages, when it is curable through hysterectomy.

HOW HRT IS ADMINISTERED

Estrogen may be taken in several different ways: orally in pills, by means of a transdermal skin patch, in a vaginal cream, or by injection (rare). Progestin is typically taken orally in pill form.

Estrogen pills, given in combination with *progestin pills*, are usually given in the following manner: one estrogen pill (0.625 milligrams each) a day for twenty-five days each month, with progestin pills (5 to 10 milligrams each) added for the last ten to fourteen days of this period, followed by five to seven days with no pills. Women on lower-dosage estrogen pills (for example, 0.3 milligrams each) should know that studies show that these lower levels offer little if any protection against osteoporosis and that the effect on heart disease is unknown.

In order to avoid the bleeding associated with HRT, another option is continuous hormone therapy, involving an estrogen pill and a low-dosage progestin pill (for example, 2.5 milligrams) each day, without any breaks.

The *transdermal skin patch* looks like a Band-Aid and is applied to the skin of the abdomen, hip, or upper thigh. It delivers estrogen directly into the bloodstream through the skin, and is changed twice a week. The patch is used for twenty-five days each month. Unlike the pill, this form of estrogen bypasses the liver and the digestive system and therefore does not have beneficial effects on cholesterol levels. Estrogen in this form is especially useful for women with liver problems that would be complicated by estrogen.

Vaginal estrogen cream is applied directly to the vagina to help counteract the dryness and loss of elasticity that many women experience during and after menopause. Its main purpose is to make sexual intercourse more comfortable. Although the estrogen in the cream is absorbed into the rest of the body through the bloodstream, the amount is too small to protect against heart disease and osteoporosis.

If you are using estrogen cream to counteract vaginal dryness and restore lubrication, apply it at least one hour before sexual intercourse. In this way, you will have given your body a chance to absorb the hormone and thus lessen the possibility that your partner will be exposed to it during intercourse.

Alternative Menopausal Treatments

Because of risk factors or negative physical reactions to HRT, not all women can use hormone replacement therapy. Others are strongly opposed to hormone use for reasons that range from the personal to the philosophical, including a conviction that the menopause is a natural phenomenon and should not be considered a medical issue.

The U.S. Congressional Office of Technology Assessment has officially approved only one nonhormonal drug for the treatment of such menopausal symptoms as hot flashes. This is Bellergal, which contains the sedative phenobarbital. Yet according to studies, Bellergal helps only about half of the women who take it and is potentially addictive.

So-called natural remedies such as vitamins and herbs, as well as certain diets, exercise, and biofeedback have not been well studied, but anecdotal reports and a few clinical investigations indicate that they may be helpful for some women. Vitamin E in daily doses of 400 to 800 International Units is one of the most popular alternative menopausal remedies. Many women who have tried it find it useful in reducing the frequency and severity of hot flashes. Vitamin B_6 in daily doses of 50 to 200 milligrams may help with various menopausal symptoms experienced by some women, such as emotional instability, tiredness, loss of libido, depression, and loss of mental concentration. However, more than 200 milligrams daily may cause neurological problems.

Ginseng contains compounds that mimic estrogen, and is available in capsules, root form, or as a tea, powder, or syrup. Its effectiveness has not been tested scientifically, but it has had a reputation as a menopausal remedy for a long time. Other foods, such as alfalfa, cherries, sesame seeds, and many others, contain plant estrogens, but there is little evidence that they are effective in combating menopausal symptoms. Biofeedback techniques for regulating body temperature may hold promise for controlling hot flashes, but such techniques have yet to be developed for this purpose.

Lastly, various drugs such as clonidine have been shown in studies to reduce the severity and frequency of hot flashes. But unpleasant side effects may occur with their use and other menopausal symptoms such as vaginal dryness and bone loss persist.

Prevention Practices

All menopausal women, regardless of whether or not they use HRT, can improve their health and lower the risk of heart disease, osteoporosis, and other health problems by the following measures:

• A diet low in fat, with adequate calcium and fiber (see Chapter 5).
• Regular exercise (see Chapter 5).
• Moderate alcohol use and no smoking.
• Stress reduction measures.
• Regular medical tests, including Pap tests and mammograms. Mammograms should be done annually throughout life after the age of fifty, for the early detection of breast cancer. (Medicare now provides reimbursement for mammograms.)
• Monthly breast self-exams.

Home Remedies for Sexual Discomfort

If you are experiencing minimal discomfort and do not wish or are unable to use hormone replacement therapy, a simple lubricant that dissolves in water (Lubrin, K-Y jelly, HR Lubricating Jelly, or Gyne-Moistrin, for example) can be placed in the vagina before intercourse to reduce dryness and friction. A moisturizing gel in tampon form called Replens, available over the counter, can be inserted vaginally three times a week to build up a continuously moist layer in the vagina. Do *not* use oil-based lubricants such as petroleum jelly, because they do not dissolve in water and can be a vehicle for vaginal infection. Remember also that the use of antihistamines and certain decongestants can dry out the mucous membranes of the vagina.

Bacterial or viral cystitis is often preventable. If you have a predisposition to infection, carefully wash the vaginal area and your partner's penis with soap and water before sexual activity to reduce the possibility. Older women should urinate before lovemaking, since a full bladder is more easily irritated. Immediately after intercourse drink large amounts of water and urinate frequently to flush out any disease agents. If your symptoms persist, seek medical care.

Wear cotton panties rather than nonabsorbent nylon or other synthetics. They can help prevent infections by allowing air to circulate in the vaginal area. For the same reason, do not wear girdles, pantyhose, and tight slacks regularly.

Since the clitoral area of older women is often more sensitive to trauma or irritation, try to ensure that your sexual partner does not touch this area in a way that produces pain. Be frank in telling your partner what is pleasurable and what is not. You may also alleviate the discomfort of honeymoon cystitis by changes in sexual positioning. The male should thrust his penis downward toward the back of the vagina and in the direction of the rectum, rather than toward the upper part of the vagina. This protects both the bladder and the delicate urethra.

The following table explains how you can modify your lifestyle to prevent the frequent occurrence of infections in the urinary tract.

PREVENTING URINARY TRACT INFECTIONS

1. Drink lots of fluid every day. Try to drink a glass of water every 2 or 3 hours.

2. Urinate frequently and try to empty your bladder completely each time. Never try to hold your urine once your bladder feels full.

---

3. Keep the bacteria in your bowels and anus away from your urethra by wiping yourself from front to back after urinating or having a bowel movement. Wash your genitals from front to back with plain water or very mild soap at least once a day.

4. Any sexual activity that irritates the urethra, puts pressure on the bladder, or spreads bacteria from the anus to the vagina or urethra can contribute to cystitis. Make sure that you and your partner have clean hands and genitals before sex, and wash after contact with the anal area before touching the vagina or urethra. To prevent irritation to the urethra, try to avoid prolonged direct clitoral stimulation and pressure on the urethral area during oral-genital sex or masturbation. Make sure your vagina is well lubricated before intercourse. Rear-entry positions and prolonged vigorous intercourse tend to put additional stress on the urethra and bladder. Emptying your bladder before and immediately after sex is a good idea. If you tend to get cystitis after sex despite these precautions, you may want to ask your practitioner for preventive tablets (e.g., sulfa, ampicillin, nitrofurantoin); a sin-

gle dose of a tablet after sex has been shown effective in preventing infections and is usually not associated with the same negative effects as a prolonged course of antibiotics.

5. Tight jeans, bicycling, or horseback riding may cause trauma to the urethra. When you engage in sports that can provoke cystitis in you, wear loose clothing and try to drink extra water.

6. Caffeine and alcohol irritate the bladder. If you don't want to stop using them, try to drink less of them and drink enough water to dilute them.

7. Some women find that routine use of cranberry juice (preferably the kind without sugar) or vitamin C to make their urine more acidic helps to prevent urinary tract problems. Whole grains, meats, nuts, and many fruits also help to acidify the urine. Avoid strong spices (curry, cayenne, chili, black pepper).

8. Diets high in refined sugars and starches (white flour, white rice, pasta, etc.) may predispose some women to urinary tract infections.

9. Keep up your resistance by eating and

resting well and finding ways to reduce stress
in your life as much as possible.

Adapted from The New Our Bodies, Ourselves *by the
Boston Women's Health Book Collective (Simon &
Schuster, 1984).*

OLDER MEN

Most men secretly begin to worry about sexual aging at
some time in their thirties, when they start to compare
their present level of sexual activity with their previous
performance as teenagers and very young adults. These
worries tend to accelerate in the forties and fifties and
reach a peak in the sixties as they continue to observe
definite sexual changes.

What changes do men notice? Quite simply, their
sexual organs don't work in the same way as they did at
a younger age. As Fred, a man in his late fifties, com-
mented: "I'm definitely slower about having an erection—and quite frankly, this is unnerving. I have been
divorced for several years, and recently on a business
trip I stopped to see a woman with whom I had had a
wonderful affair some twenty years ago. We found we
were still attracted to each other. But when we at-

tempted to make love, it took me forever to get things underway. She took this as a sign that I wasn't interested in her, and we ended up not having sex at all. I was totally humiliated and so was she. What a disaster!"

Lacking a full understanding of this change, men misinterpret it as alarming, and as either the onset of impotence or its future inevitability. "From a psycho-sexual point of view," say Masters and Johnson, "the male over age fifty has to contend with one of the great fallacies of our culture. Every man in this age group is arbitrarily identified by both public and professional alike as sexually impaired."

Potency is the man's sexual capacity for inter-course. Impotence is the temporary or permanent in-capacity to have an erection sufficient to carry out the sexual act. (Do not confuse sterility with impotence. Sterility means infertility or the incapacity to father chil-dren.) What is normal potency for one man may not be normal for another. There are variations in the fre-quency of erection and the length of time a man main-tains an erection. Such individual differences often continue over many years, defining unique personal pat-terns. Therefore comparisons of a man's present sexual status must be made in terms of *his* past history and not in terms of some generalized "standard" involving com-parisons with other men. Most sex therapists do not consider impotence or erectile dysfunction to be a prob-lem unless it occurs in 25 percent or more of sexual encounters with the same partner.

While individual variation from man to man must be taken into account, there are a number of gradual and fairly predictable processes which affect sexuality that are associated with chronological aging. An older man ordinarily takes longer to obtain an erection than a younger man. The difference is a matter of minutes after sexual stimulation rather than a few seconds. The erection may also not be quite as large, straight, and hard as in previous years. Once the man is fully excited, however, his erection will usually be sturdy and reliable, particularly if this was the pattern in earlier life. A critical point to remember is that increased manual stimulation of the penis by the man himself or his partner is often helpful in promoting and maintaining arousal.

The lubrication that appears prior to ejaculation (Cowper's gland secretory activity) decreases or disappears completely as men age, but this has little effect on sexual performance. There is also a reduction in the volume of seminal fluid, and this results in a decrease in the need to ejaculate. Younger men produce 3 to 5 milliliters of semen (about one teaspoon) every twenty-four hours, while men past fifty produce 2 to 3 milliliters. This can be a decided advantage in lovemaking, since it means that the older man can delay ejaculation more easily and thus make love longer, extending his own enjoyment and enhancing the possibility of orgasm for his partner.

Even orgasms may begin to feel different with age. The younger man is aware of a few pleasurable seconds, just before ejaculation, when he can no longer control himself. As ejaculation occurs, powerful contractions are felt and the semen spurts with a force that can carry it one to two feet from the tip of the penis. With an older man there may be a briefer period of awareness before ejaculation or no such period at all. (In some men, however, this period actually lengthens because of spasms in the prostate.) The orgasm itself is generally less explosive, in that the semen is propelled a shorter distance and the contractions are less forceful. *None* of these physiological changes interferes with the aging man's experiencing extreme orgasmic pleasure, even when the pre-ejaculation stage is altered or completely missing.

The forcefulness of orgasm also lessens naturally when a couple voluntarily prolong their lovemaking before orgasm. Many older men become aware that they have a choice of an extended period of sexual pleasure with a milder orgasm or a briefer session with a more intense orgasm.

Whereas younger men can usually have another ejaculation in a matter of minutes after orgasm, the older man generally must wait a longer period of time (the refractory period), from several hours up to several days, before an ejaculation is again possible. In addition, the older man may rapidly lose his erection following orgasm, sometimes so quickly that the penis literally slips out of the vagina. This is not a sign of impairment of the penis and its erectile capacity, but simply a physical change that requires a mental adjustment.

Older men should not fall into the common trap of measuring manhood by the frequency with which they can carry intercourse through to ejaculation. Some men over sixty are physically satisfied with one or two ejaculations per week because of the decrease of semen production. Others, particularly if they were less sexually active earlier in life, do not ejaculate this frequently. Each man should find a level of ejaculatory frequency he is comfortable with. Remember that lovemaking need not be limited to ejaculatory ability. Men who are knowledgeable and comfortable about themselves may have intercourse as frequently as they wish but ejaculate perhaps only once out of every two or three times that they make love. By delaying ejaculation, an older man may be able to become erect over and over again, continuing with intercourse and the pleasurable feelings it arouses.

Male fertility—sperm production—generally ends in the midseventies, though there have been instances where it continued into the nineties. A urologist can test for the presence of live sperm through a microscopic examination of semen. Again, *fertility has no connection with potency* (erectile capacity); even if a man loses his capacity to father children, his ability to have intercourse is not affected by loss of sperm production.

In general, men do *not* lose their capacity to have erections and ejaculations as they age. The patterns of sexual activity of healthy men as they grow older tend to reflect earlier patterns in their lives, with the added factor of a somewhat slower physical response due to aging. Problems that may occur, particularly impotence, are caused by physical or psychological difficulties; frequently they are treatable.

In fact, according to current studies, interest in sex or sexual desire is believed to decline only slightly with age in healthy men. And that desire does not necessarily change even in those who experience a loss of erectile capacity or a change in orgasmic frequency. It is the amount of sexual activity itself, besides a decrease in ejaculatory amount, that does tend to decrease. Some speculate that this may be influenced by changes in the central nervous system that reduce the male's ability to translate visual sexual stimuli into physical arousal. Other factors may be disease processes under way but not yet obvious.

Finally, the unavailability of one's mate obviously has an impact upon the amount of sexual activity. Ninety-one-year-old Henry, who lost his wife a number of years earlier, wrote to us:

> I have been "on the shelf," as they say, for the past four years—no more sex, just thinking about it, which is not sufficient. If I could find a lady friend who would accept a guy in a wheelchair, I might give it another try.

IS THERE A MALE MENOPAUSE?

Do men experience a period in life that is physically or psychologically comparable to a female's cessation of menstruation and loss of estrogen hormones? There is certainly no physical "menopause" or climacteric in men that is analogous to that in women, because hormone loss in men does not occur precipitously. (Actually, hormone loss in women occurs in spurts, never in a single, abrupt cessation.) Decreases in the male hormone testosterone take place very gradually—if at all—with age, and it fluctuates widely from man to man. Some older men actually have testosterone levels identical with those in young men. And few men have specific physiological symptoms that can be traced directly to lowered testosterone levels. In a few uncommon cases, as with Perry, men do experience some physical problems.

Perry thought that his difficulties in obtaining an erection at the age of sixty-nine were a sign of "aging" and that it was all over for him when it came to sexual matters. He was more or less accepting of his fate. His wife, however, insisted on his seeing a doctor. She had to be incredibly persistent, for he was extremely reluctant to seek medical advice. Fortunately, it was discovered that his condition was among the rare instances of primary hypogonadism, which is low levels of testosterone. Through the artificial administration of testosterone he was soon able to achieve an erection.

Distinct psychological symptoms are also rare when male hormone loss occurs, and can usually be accounted for by other circumstances in a man's life, such as his reactions to retirement, to aging in general, or to other stresses.

As research on male hormone levels becomes more sophisticated and reliable, it may eventually be possible to define a male climacteric, or as some have called it, "andropause," particularly in terms of some of the sexual changes that accompany male aging. However, it will be quite different from our concept of female menopause, with far less distinct and less predictable symptoms.

Physical Sexual Changes—Are They Aging or Disease?

We do not yet know whether all the physiological changes we have described in this chapter are "normal aging" processes or symptoms of reversible physical conditions. The fact that a man takes longer to achieve an erection as he gets older, or requires a longer period of time before an erection can occur again after the last sexual act, may possibly be related to reduced nutritive, oxygen, and blood supplies resulting from hardening of the arteries (arteriosclerosis). From a variety of studies we know that much of the physical change attributed to aging is in fact due to a variety of other factors, notably the vascular diseases. The integrative systems of the body that link so many of its functions—the circulatory system, the endocrine (or hormonal) system, the central nervous system—all play a role in the decline of functioning when they are affected by diseases. We are only beginning to have some knowledge of the fundamentals of the aging process itself: Is there a central-nervous-system pacemaker that dictates change? Are there reductions in the speed of reactions and in metabolism?

It is possible that in the future we will find that sexual activity among older people actually improves as we increasingly separate out the diseases and psychological impairments of old age from the aging processes, and begin to prevent and treat them. Furthermore, if aging factors become more clear-cut and if agents that work to retard the process of aging are found, there will be still further changes in the sexual picture. What relatively healthy men and women need to remember, even under the limitations of our present knowledge about aging, is that sexual activity—to whatever degree and in whatever forms they want to express it—should continue to be possible, normal, pleasurable, and beneficial. Those older people with fairly common chronic ailments can, in many cases, adapt their sexual desires so that they can find some kind of satisfactory expression. Remember: neither age nor in most cases infirmity automatically spells the end of sex.

CHAPTER 3

❧❧❧

COMMON MEDICAL
PROBLEMS AND HOW
THEY AFFECT
LOVEMAKING

ILLNESS AND SEX

What happens to one's sexuality when illness strikes? An acute illness that is sudden and severe has an immediate effect. The body becomes totally involved in meeting the physical threat, and anxiety is strong until the crisis has passed and the full extent of the illness is known. Understandably, people in these circumstances have little or no energy and attention left for sexual feelings. Once the acute phase of an illness is over, most people return slowly to sexuality; but if recovery time is lengthy or if the illness results in a chronic condition, which must be lived with, there can be problems. In this chapter we will discuss several of the more common conditions that may directly affect sexuality in people over sixty.

HEART DISEASE

Men from forty-five to sixty have heart disease at nearly three times the rate of women in this age group. After sixty the rates become more equal; it is believed the postmenopausal woman gradually becomes more vulnerable because of the reduction in her estrogen levels.

Heart (coronary) attacks lead many people to give up sex altogether under the assumption that it will endanger their lives. Recent studies show that many couples decrease or stop all sexual activity after a heart attack, often because their doctors haven't given them adequate advice about sex. Studies also show that the person who does resume sexual activity usually waits about sixteen weeks, with those who had the most active sex lives before a coronary resuming their sex lives the soonest. Many experts believe that an eight-to-fourteen-week waiting period is an adequate amount of time before resuming lovemaking; of course, it all depends on the patient's desire, general fitness, and conditioning. Self-stimulation or mutual masturbation can be an alternative to sex, and it can usually be started earlier than sexual intercourse. Some doctors propose a simple functional test to determine when it is safe to resume sex: If you can walk briskly for three blocks without distress in the chest, pain, palpitations, or shortness of breath, you are usually well enough for sexual exertion.

Sex *can* be carried out safely without sacrificing pleasure and quality. Studies tell us that, on the average, couples take ten to sixteen minutes for the sex act. The oxygen usage (or "cost") in sex is approximately equal to climbing one or two flights of stairs, walking rapidly at a rate of two to two and a half miles an hour, or completing many common occupational tasks. In average sexual activity the heart rate ranges from 90 to 160 beats a minute, which is the level for light to moderate physical activity. Systolic blood pressure (the upper reading, which reflects the contraction phase of the heart's action) may double, from 120 to over 240, and the respiratory rate rises from sixteen or eighteen to about sixty breaths a minute. These vital signs increase slightly more in men than in women, perhaps due in part to the usual sexual position of the man on top. If the man is the one with the heart problem, conduct intercourse side by side or with the woman on top to reduce his exertion. These positions avoid the sapping of energy that occurs after a prolonged use of the arms and legs to support the body. Proper physical conditioning (usually a program of brisk walking and/or swimming) under a doctor's guidance can also be useful, in part because such conditioning can lower the pulse-rate rise during sex.

Physical-fitness programs can enhance heart performance for a variety of activities, including sex. Isometric exercises, however, may be unwise for certain people because they cause pressure changes in the aorta, the major blood vessel from the heart, so be sure to check with your physician. Before undertaking an exercise program, ask your doctor to arrange special testing in which an electrocardiogram, or EKG (a tracing of the heart's electric currents that provides information regarding the heart's actions in health and disease), is taken while you engage in exercise at various intensities. An electromagnetic tape recording of your EKG during the sexual act can even be made in your own home. This is called Hellerstein's Sexercise Tolerance Test. Drs. H. E. Hellerstein and E. H. Friedman studied the sexual activity of men after recovery from an acute heart attack by monitoring sexual activities in the privacy of their patients' homes. They reported that if the men could perform exercise at levels of vigorous walking and other special activities without symptoms of abnormal pulse rate, blood pressure, or EKG changes, it was generally safe for them to resume sexual activity.

Some physicians warn, though, that such stress tests are not infallible. They can produce false alarms for healthy people, while in other cases coronary disease may not be detected. A medical and sexual history, the patient's report concerning any chest pain he or she may experience during exertion, and a resting EKG should all be part of the stress test.

Please remember that physical exercise leads to less likelihood of a heart attack. The sedentary person may be more prone to coronary attacks and less apt to survive the experience if one occurs. Too much food and drink before sexual intercourse can also place a strain on the heart. Of course, if the condition of the heart has deteriorated to the point that an attack is imminent, it will occur with any physical exertion, not merely sex. In fact, sexual intercourse may produce less increase in heart and respiratory rates than many everyday nonsexual activities.

It should also be realized that sexual arousal alone (without intercourse) affects the vital signs (although not as intensely as the sexual act itself). Failure to provide sexual release may prolong arousal, causing a psychological frustration that may produce some adverse physical effects.

Potency problems can follow a heart attack for both physical and psychological reasons. A man may then experience chest pain (angina pectoris) during various forms of exertion, including sex, that frightens him and thus prevents erection. To counteract this pain, take coronary dilators such as nitroglycerin, prescribed by a physician, to improve circulation and reduce the pain just prior to intercourse. A second common—and quite understandable—cause of impotence is fear of inducing another coronary and risking death. This was the case with Frank.

Frank, age seventy-two, used to be amused by the fact that the French phrase for sexual orgasm is *petite mort* (little death). But it no longer seemed as funny after he had his heart attack and became obsessed with the thought that he might die from the exertion of sexual intercourse. It became virtually impossible for him to initiate sexual activity with his wife. She was puzzled and saddened by his remoteness, and finally insisted that they both see his heart doctor. Since Frank was too embarrassed to bring up the subject, she told the doctor what was wrong: her husband was scaring himself into sexual inactivity. The doctor reassured both of them that Frank was in good enough physical condition to engage in any level of lovemaking. She demonstrated this by putting Frank on a treadmill and showing him the levels of physical exertion he could handle with no sign of overstress on his heart. Frank and his wife were greatly relieved and quickly returned to their usual patterns of sexuality.

In fact, the incidence of death during intercourse is estimated at less that 1 percent. (In one major study the rate was less than 0.3 percent!) Of this small percentage, seven out of ten deaths occur in extramarital relations, suggesting that it is the stressful aspects associated with such affairs—i.e., guilt, anxiety, the need to hurry—that may play a role.

Feeling depressed and anxious after a heart attack is common. You may also feel irritable and exhausted, and you might believe that your partner is no longer attracted to you. Conversely, your partner may become overly protective and fearful of upsetting you. In most cases, these are just normal reactions to what has been a tremendously frightening experience, and they will subside in time. If they do not, consider talking about these feelings with a physician or psychotherapist so that they do not harm your relationship or sex life.

Physicians, however, do not always advise their patients adequately on how and when to resume sexual activity after a heart attack. If you want to know more than your doctor has told you, it may be necessary to ask for specific information and directions, including a program of physical conditioning. Your partner also needs to be fully informed and counseled about any changes in life-style, and specifically lovemaking, that may be necessary. *Under most circumstances there is little reason to abstain from sex after a heart attack, and many reasons to continue!* You may experience pleasure, exhilaration, release of tension, mild exercise, and a sense of well-being. However, after resuming sexual activity, you should report any of the following occurrences to your doctor: (1) anginal pain occurring during or after sex; (2) palpitations continuing for fifteen minutes or more afterward; (3) unusual episodes of sleeplessness after sexual exertion; and (4) marked fatigue the next day.

To alleviate any potential stress during periods of lovemaking, it helps to: (1) have a familiar and considerate partner; (2) wait three hours or more after eating or drinking alcohol; (3) use a room with a moderate temperature; and (4) choose a relaxed time, such as the morning after a restful night. If you begin to feel strained or anxious during lovemaking, simply stop and breathe deeply for a few minutes before beginning again.

Episodes of congestive heart failure are also commonly called heart attacks. When they are compensated for by digitalis, diuretics, and diet, having sex is again an active possibility. However, it is advisable to wait two to three weeks before having sex again.

Those with cardiac pacemakers need not give up sex unless the condition of their heart precludes such activity. But you should limit all forms of physical activity during the first two weeks following the implantation to allow for healing. The guidelines to follow will vary, based on your doctor's evaluation of the underlying cardiac condition.

Coronary Bypass Surgery

Because of actual symptoms, the treatment of this disease, or the fear of sudden death from sexual activity, many people have some kind of sexual dysfunction by the time they have coronary bypass surgery. After the surgery, you must learn what level of activity you can undertake without stressing your chest bones. Most of you will be advised to walk and move about very soon after the surgery. For those who fear the resumption of lovemaking, it may be reassuring to embark on exercise programs that improve heart capacity; this is what Ted, seventy-two, did after his bypass.

Ted had always been physically active: He was a runner, then a jogger, and more recently a fast walker. But his genetic background worked against him. He had a high level of cholesterol despite his excellent program of physical fitness and his diet, which stresses low fat and low cholesterol. His own view, which is shared by his doctor, is that had he not engaged in a vigorous physical and dietary program, he might not be alive today. Recently he had his first coronary bypass operation. It was his desire to continue his sex life that motivated him to make a quick return to his previous level of physical fitness. He visits the Pritikin Longevity Center annually to monitor his physical status, learn the latest diet and exercise techniques for his particular condition, and motivate himself to "stay on the program." As of this writing Ted has continued to stay healthy.

Many form a psychological dependence on taking nitroglycerin, a drug that alleviates chest pain, before having sex, even though surgery may have eliminated the need for it. To rid yourself of this dependency, obtain support from others who have successfully weaned themselves from nitroglycerin, or failing this, have your doctor prescribe a mild antianxiety medication for a brief time.

Those who require medications such as beta blockers, which can decrease sexual desire and cause impotence, may be able to switch to other medications with fewer sexual side effects, such as calcium blockers like verapamil. Those with arrhythmias (irregular heartbeat) that do not require treatment need reassurance and perhaps a heart monitor (the Holter monitor) or a treadmill test to calm anxiety about sexual activity. In some cases antiarrhythmic drugs and beta blockers cannot be avoided; if this happens to you, bear in mind that such drugs are life-protective, and if they interfere with your sexual desire and performance, you can and should concentrate on other forms of intimacy and physical pleasure.

In sum, then, many coronary bypass surgery patients can expect to return to a reasonable level of sexual activity. An exercise and nutritional program can improve your chances. *Short-term* treatment of anxiety and depression with the appropriate drugs can be helpful in leading toward the resumption of lovemaking, but in the long run you will find counseling, psychotherapy, and information about heart attacks to be more effective treatment methods. *Heartmates—A Survival Guide for the Cardiac Spouse* by Rhoda Levin (Prentice-Hall, 1987) offers sound advice.

HYPERTENSION

It is safe for most people with hypertension—high blood pressure—to have sex. (Many with hypertension have no significant impairment of heart function at all.) As a general rule, then, those with average to moderate hypertension need not restrict themselves sexually. You should, however, have your hypertension well controlled by diet, physical exercise, and, when appropriate, drug therapy. If you have very severe hypertension it may be best to modify your sexual activity; your doctor can best judge this.

Men with untreated hypertension are reported to have about a 15 percent incidence of impotence. Such sexual impairment can be avoided by properly treating the hypertension; weight loss if one is overweight (especially through the reduction of fat and sugar intake), regular exercise, reduction of cholesterol and triglyceride levels, limitation of salt to five grams or less a day, moderate use of alcohol, and no smoking are the first steps in treatment. Biofeedback therapies are also effective for some. If these do not bring your blood pressure down to acceptable levels, you will need medication. Such medication must be carefully chosen to avoid side effects of impaired sexual response (see page 112).

STROKE

Unless a stroke (cerebrovascular accident) causes severe trauma to the brain, sexual desire often continues; it is the physical performance that is more likely to be affected, especially in the earlier periods following the stroke. Men tend to have erectile and ejaculatory difficulty, while women may experience problems with vaginal lubrication.

However, strokes do not demand that all sexual activity cease. Even if paralysis has occurred, appropriate sexual positions often can be found to compensate for it. When choosing a treatment plan make sure that sexual rehabilitation is an important component of it. You and your partner may find it helpful to refer to S. Burgener's "Sexuality Concerns of the Post-Stroke Patient" in *Rehabilitation Nursing*, July–August 1989 (this journal is available in many medical libraries). It is also important to make note of the fact that sexual activity has *not* been found to be a factor in bringing on a stroke or in causing more damage to those who have had a stroke.

DIABETES

Sugar diabetes (diabetes mellitus) is a common occurrence in late life. Most men with diabetes are *not* impotent, but it *is* one of the few illnesses that can directly cause chronic impotence in men. Impotence occurs two to five times as often in diabetics as in the general population, and is often the first symptom of diabetes.

In most cases of diabetes-produced impotence, sexual interest and desire are not affected, and the impotence itself is reversible. There is a fair chance when the diabetes is poorly controlled that upon proper regulation, potency will improve. This was the case with sixty-two-year-old Barry, who had his moderate diabetes under poor control.

Barry was a heavy smoker (two or more packs daily), and his travel schedule made good nutrition and proper exercise problematic. Barry suffered from both financial and marital troubles, and for him, all sexual activity had ceased. Luckily for Barry, his doctor insisted that Barry enter a treatment program where he was placed on a low-fat diet with carefully monitored amounts of physical exercise. Three weeks later his diabetes was under control and Barry had learned how to adapt his fitness program so that he could continue it while on business travel. And (this impressed him the most) his sexual capacity returned to him in full force.

There is a percentage of cases of diabetes in which the impotence is not reversible; unfortunately, when impotence occurs in well-controlled diabetes it may well be permanent. And if you have been diabetic for a long time, the chances are greater that the impotence will be chronic and irreversible.

With women it is more difficult to evaluate the effects of diabetes on sexuality, since women do not have an obvious physical indicator like erection. However, current research strongly suggests that sexuality is affected far less by diabetes in women than in men.

CANCER

Although one out of every four Americans is expected to develop some form of cancer in his or her lifetime, survival rates are improving and many people who have had bouts of cancer go on to live normal lives. However, the effects of cancer and its treatment can have a negative impact on sexual functioning. We will be discussing several examples in the next chapter. But because of the many different kinds of cancers and the complexity of cancer treatment, if the effects of cancer on sexuality are an issue for you, we recommend two excellent booklets by Leslie R. Schover, Ph.D., titled *Sexuality and Cancer: For the Woman Who Has Cancer and Her Partner* and *Sexuality and Cancer: For the Man Who Has Cancer and His Partner* (1988), available from the American Cancer Society.

CHRONIC PROSTATITIS

Diminished sexual desire in men may be associated with chronic prostatitis. This disease is an inflammation of the prostate gland, a walnut-sized organ located just beneath the bladder in the male. It produces the milky lubricating fluid that transports sperm during sexual intercourse. You may experience pain in the perineal region (the area between the scrotum and the anus) and in the end of the penis on urination and ejaculation, and find that manual manipulation of the prostate causes tenderness. Treatment for such a condition includes antibiotics, warm sitz baths, and periodic gentle prostatic massage by a physician. Sexual desire usually returns after the pain lessens—especially when the pain after ejaculation is eliminated.

Many doctors believe that some cases of nonbacterial prostatitis are caused by both too frequent and too infrequent sex. The basis for some pain between the anus and the scrotum after ejaculation may be mild prostatitis; other causes are congestion due to excessive or lengthy preliminary sexual arousal, or an unsatisfying orgasm. However, a more common cause is infrequent sex, which results in congestion in the pelvic area. Treatment in these cases consists of more frequent ejaculation as well as prostatic massage and warm sitz baths. Some believe that the practice of Kegel exercises (see pages 151–152) may help.

If you have chronic prostatitis, avoid the intake of excessive alcohol. Urinary retention can occasionally develop following sexual intercourse; this may be caused by the combination of a large fluid intake and the sedative effect of alcohol. If there is also some enlargement of the prostate without inflammation, excessive fluid intake, including alcohol, may lead to retention of urine.

ARTHRITIS

Arthritis is a widespread condition that affects forty million Americans and strikes women twice as often as men. Rheumatoid arthritis, commonly beginning between ages twenty-five and fifty, and osteoarthritis, a later-life condition, are the two major forms of arthritis and may cause pain during sexual activity. Medications such as simple aspirin are used to reduce pain. It is reassuring to know that most drugs used to treat arthritis, except for corticosteroids, do not interfere with either sexual desire or sexual performance. You might also experiment with new sexual positions that do not aggravate pain in those joints that are sensitive. A well-established program of exercise, rest, and warm baths works wonders at reducing arthritic discomfort and facilitating sex. Indeed, much of the crippling effect of rheumatoid arthritis results from inactivity; a person tends to keep painful joints in comfortable positions, and they become stiffened, even "frozen." For information on exercise and other treatments, write for the free publication list published by the Arthritis Foundation, 67 Irving Place, New York, NY 10003, or call 212-477-8700. Several reprints dealing specifically with sexuality and arthritis are also available from them.

Hip discomfort is perhaps the most frequent arthritic problem to affect sexual activity directly. Hip action during sex may be slowed down or made difficult because of pain or changes in the ability to move the hips. When the problem is severe, many choose surgical hip replacement, which may restore function, including that involved in sex. For less severe conditions, a range of therapies can be beneficial. Exercise, prescribed by your doctor, should include a full range of motion for the joints, strengthening and stretching of muscles, and engaging in the usual household and outside activities. You should also maintain an erect position when standing and walking, sit upright in a straight-backed chair, and rest in bed for short periods several times during the day. In general, rest or sleep in a straight position, flat on the back, using a small pillow under the head (a pillow under the knees can lead to stiff, bent knees).

The use of heat, both before undertaking an exercise program and prior to sex, relaxes any muscle spasms. Feel free to use various types of heat—heat lamps, heating pads, warm compresses, tub baths, showers, and paraffin baths. A daily tub bath with warm, not hot, water that lasts for no more than twenty minutes is excellent (longer baths can be fatiguing). You may also find that a water bed and massage oils may enhance your comfort. During lovemaking you may find that the side-by-side position—either face-to-face or back-to-front—is preferable, especially if you or your partner has tender areas and pain trigger points. As always, experiment until you find the positions that work best for you. Bear in mind that pillows can help in cushioning painful joints.

Timing can also be important. Some discover that pain and stiffness diminish or disappear completely at certain times of the day, so plan lovemaking for these times. Max and Molly, both in their early seventies, discovered the importance of this after retiring and settling in Florida. Their happiness at being retired and at having plenty of time for their personal relationship ran into snags, particularly with regard to their sex life. Molly has severe osteoarthritis, which gets worse at the end of the day. In particular, Molly has a great deal of discomfort in her hips. Together she and her husband consulted a sensitive and sympathetic internist, who encouraged them to take advantage of their retirement time and engage in lovemaking in the morning, after a good night's rest. This was the most pain-free time for Molly. Plus, it was suggested that they use the side-by-side sexual position, which puts less physical pressure on Molly. Even before beginning sexual activity, they found that a long, hot shower helped Molly relax physically. To further diminish her pain, she was advised to take aspirin and use pillows to cushion her hip bones.

All of this enabled the couple to moderate and even eliminate Molly's arthritic pain. Furthermore, their time together became more intimate and tender than it had ever been at its best in their earlier years, because Molly was so touched by Max's concern for her.

Those who suffer from osteoarthritis, like Molly, will usually find morning to be the best part of the day, with discomfort increasing at the end of the day, while those with rheumatoid arthritis usually feel greater pain and stiffness in the morning. Be sure to ask your doctor to time pain or anti-inflammatory medications so they will be most effective at times when you are most likely to have sexual activity. A condition known as Sjögren's syndrome occurs with some forms of arthritis and results in a decrease in body secretions. A lubricant such as K-Y jelly will compensate for inadequate vaginal secretions.

Indeed, it may be physically beneficial for arthritis sufferers to engage in sex. Evidence suggests that regular sexual activity may produce some relief from the pain of rheumatoid arthritis for four to eight hours, probably because of adrenal gland production of the hormone cortisone and because of the physical activity involved. The body's release of endorphins, its natural pain relievers, during sexual activity and especially during orgasm may also be a factor. Finally, emotional stress can result from sexual dissatisfaction, and since stress worsens arthritis, satisfying sexual activity can be helpful in maintaining a healthy and pain-free body.

BACKACHE

Backache in the small of the back near the base of the spine is extremely common among older people. It is frequently caused by a generally inactive person suddenly using the back muscles and placing strain on the back. In women the backache can also be traced to osteoporosis (postmenopausal thinning of the bones), which is related to the reduction in estrogen levels. Slipped discs and arthritis also cause backaches in both men and women.

Most backache sufferers need a firm mattress and bed board. A plywood board at least one-half inch thick and the same size as the mattress can be placed between the mattress and springs for extra support. Exercise is helpful for most forms of backache, but you should see your doctor and exercise therapist for instructions in your particular case. While slipped discs often respond well to exercise, sometimes they may require prolonged bed rest; otherwise, surgery may be necessary. Those who suffer from arthritic backache should follow the program described above for arthritis.

Sexual activity itself is an excellent form of exercise therapy for the back, stomach, and pelvic muscles, and if undertaken in a regular and reasonably vigorous manner, can help reduce back pain. During sex, you may find that the side position is the most comfortable if your back muscles are tender. Or you may prefer lying on your back, with your partner on top. Again, remember to support areas of discomfort with pillows.

ANEMIA

One out of four people over sixty has some measure of anemia, a common cause of fatigue and consequent reduction of sexual activity. Anemia may develop insidiously following even a mild general or localized infection, or as a result of a poor diet. Tiredness, loss of appetite, and headaches are some of its early symptoms. Since anemia is the symptom of a number of diseases, a comprehensive medical examination is needed. Follow-up treatment is extremely important. Often an improved diet with adequate vitamins and minerals is all that is necessary to restore both energy and sexual activity.

CHRONIC CYSTITIS AND URETHRITIS

Some women experience recurrent outbreaks of cystitis and urethritis following intercourse. The chief symptoms are severe pain and burning around the urethra. Yet the cause is often unclear, and if no organisms can be found in their urine, women are often told their problem is psychological. What this can lead to is outrage at the doctor, feelings of depression, continued pain, and a sense of hopelessness.

Do not give up even if you have to undergo a long diagnostic process until the cause or causes are found and corrected. Surgical correction, medications, education on sexual techniques and positions, pain management, and interpersonal counseling are all possible avenues of treatment, depending on your physician's recommendation. And your sexual partner should be checked for possible untreated prostatitis. Plus, you must deal with the depression that usually accompanies chronic cystitis. Above all, your physician should persist in searching for the cause, and you should not be told it is all in your head. Take comfort in the fact that even long-standing cystitis can be evaluated and cured.

STRESS OR URGE INCONTINENCE

Nearly one woman in five over the age of forty will develop stress incontinence (caused by stretched pelvic muscles), a condition in which there is an involuntary seepage of urine because of a momentary inability to control the bladder. This happens particularly when you laugh, cough, engage in sex, or otherwise exert yourself. Urge incontinence is a sudden, painful urge to void (or no sensation at all) before you can get to a bathroom. Sexual dysfunction of various sorts has been reported in up to 50 percent of women with this condition. In fact, you might even experience dyspareunia, or painful intercourse. Stress incontinence is most frequently seen in women who have had a number of children and who might have unrepaired injuries following a birth, resulting in a relaxation of the uterine and bladder supports.

Obesity and estrogen deficiency can also be strongly associated with the occurrence of this kind of incontinence. It is also seen in women who have had the uterus removed surgically (hysterectomy) or who have slack supporting tissues that may cause the bladder to protrude into the vagina (cystocele). Inserting a large tampon in the vagina, which gives support to the bladder, can sometimes provide temporary relief. To guard against toxic shock syndrome, do not leave the tampon in place for more than a few hours. Estrogen taken by mouth or applied locally in the form of a cream may help firm up the vaginal lining and thus reduce the irritation that may develop from the protruding bladder. You can also engage in specialized exercises, called Kegel exercises (described on pages 151–152), to strengthen the muscles that support the bladder. Weight loss may also have a positive impact on this condition. If the incontinence persists, you can purchase a wide variety of pads that provide hygiene security.

Biofeedback training may also improve the incontinence. In the most severe cases, you may require surgery to reposition the internal pelvic organs and tighten the muscles. Such surgery can be done under local or spinal anesthesia, and its success rate is very high.

A self-help and advocacy organization called HIP (Help for Incontinent People) can provide information and lists of resources. Write to HIP, P.O. Box 544, Union, SC 29379, and include a business-size self-addressed stamped envelope. HIP will provide a list of its many helpful and informative publications on incontinence, as well as information about its quarterly newsletter, *The HIP Report*. You may also wish to purchase HIP's *Resource Guide of Continence Products and Services* as well as audio- and videotapes.

The Association for Urinary Continence Control, 785 Park Avenue, New York, NY 10021 (212-988-8888), offers a multispecialty approach for male and female patients suffering from urinary incontinence. The group includes an internist, a psychiatrist, a gynecologist, a urologist, and others who will work together to diagnose and treat incontinence in an integrated manner. Continence Restored, Inc., 785 Park Avenue, New York, NY 10021, will send information on current support groups and how to form a support group. The Simon Foundation, P.O. Box 815, Wilmette, IL 60091 (phone: 800-23-SIMON), will provide information, a free copy of its quarterly newsletter, *The Informer*, and a sample *Attends* undergarment that protects against urine leakage.

Herniation, or prolapse of the uterus and of the rectum (rectocele), may occur alone or in association with prolapse of the bladder. In this case surgical treatment is usually effective. Stress incontinence is also occasionally seen in men following prostatectomy (see page 138).

In general, doctors agree that most stress or urge incontinence can be well controlled or even totally eliminated with the proper diagnosis and treatment. However, one of the greatest frustrations women voice is a lack of support and information from urologists and other physicians when they report their incontinence problem. Be persistent and insist that your physician take action.

PARKINSON'S DISEASE

Parkinson's disease is a progressive nervous-system disorder of the later years marked by tremor, slowness of movement, partial facial paralysis, and peculiarity of posture and gait. Depression is commonly associated with Parkinson's disease and may lead to impotence in men and lack of sexual interest in both sexes. When there is advanced organic involvement, however, impotence may be physically connected with the disease.

Those with Parkinson's disease who are treated with drugs such as L-dopa may show improved sexual performance, largely because of an increased sense of well-being and greater mobility.

PEYRONIE'S DISEASE

This disorder, found in men, produces an upward bowing of the penis with the shaft angled to the right or left. A fibrous thickening of the walls of the blood vessels (corpora cavernosa) of the penis produces the symptoms, but its cause is unknown. Sometimes, after four years or so, the symptoms disappear spontaneously. Yet the results of treatment are not predictable. One therapy is the taking of p-aminobenzoate (in the form of Potaba or Potaba Plus) for about six months. For some the application of ultrasound to the fibrous areas of the penis in order to disrupt fibrous tissue has been successful, and this is especially true with those who have not had the problem for long. Surgical removal of the plaque is often successful. Cortisone is sometimes effective, but it must be injected rather than taken orally. There is no evidence that vitamin E works.

Intercourse can be painful and, if the penis is angled too far, impossible. However, in most cases of Peyronie's disease, sex can continue. This ailment is thought to be rare, but our own experience in talking with physicians and patients leads us to suspect that it may be more common than is believed.

PELVIC STEAL SYNDROME

The pelvic steal syndrome is an example of vascular impotence. In this condition the male loses his erection as soon as he enters his partner and begins pelvic thrusting. This impotence results from gravity's redirecting the blood supply from the penis to the muscles in the buttocks, which had been activated by the thrusting. To successfully overcome the pelvic steal syndrome, men should lie on their backs while making love, thus reversing the flow of gravity. A side position may work as well.

CHRONIC RENAL DISEASE

Those with chronic renal disease experience a continuum of treatments that may end with renal dialysis or renal transplants. This can be a stressful disease and is often associated with depression and anxiety. Male chronic renal patients are often sterile and may have reduced levels of serum testosterone. Other organic factors that affect one's sexuality may be present, although they have not been identified. Nonetheless, not all renal patients have sexual problems, and those who do may be treatable if the problems are not strictly organic in nature. Treating the anxiety and the depression and engaging in marital counseling can successfully combat this disorder. Kidney transplants can often restore sexual capacity.

CHRONIC EMPHYSEMA AND BRONCHITIS

Chronic emphysema and bronchitis, which entail short-ness of breath, often hinder physical activity, and that can include sex. The extent of the limitation depends on the severity of the disease. You'll find that resting at intervals and finding the least physically taxing ways to make love can help.

HERNIA OR RUPTURE

A hernia or rupture is the protrusion of a part of the intestine through a gap or weak point in the muscular abdominal wall that contains it. The main complication to avoid is strangulation, or a cutting off of the blood supply with the resulting death of tissue, which is a true surgical emergency. Straining of any kind, including straining during sexual intercourse, can sometimes in-crease hernia symptoms such as pain and, rarely, induce strangulation. Many surgeons recommend corrective surgery early on, rather than waiting for an emergency to arise.

IN SUMMARY

If you have had to abstain from sex for a medical reason for any length of time, some readjustment will be necessary when you resume sexual activity. Irregular or infrequent sexual stimulation can interfere with healthy sexual functioning, adversely affecting potency in men and lubrication, vaginal shape, and muscle tone in women. These difficulties are likely to taper off as activity is resumed, so do not be discouraged by the initial difficulties. When a sexual partner is not available or circumstances do not permit contact with a partner, both men and women can protect much of their sexual capacity through regular self-stimulation (masturbation) if this is acceptable and comfortable for them.

SEXUALLY TRANSMITTED DISEASES AND LOVEMAKING

ACQUIRED IMMUNE DEFICIENCY SYNDROME

AIDS is a condition believed to be caused by a virus called HIV (Human Immunodeficiency Virus). The virus attacks the immune system, the body's "security force" that fights off infections. When the immune system breaks down, we lose this protection and can develop many serious, often deadly infections and cancers. These are called opportunistic infections because they take advantage of the body's weakened defenses. By far the greatest number of deaths associated with AIDS are caused by a virulent type of pneumonia known as PCP (pneumocystis carnii pneumonia).

HIV can be transmitted through certain body fluids: blood, semen, vaginal secretions, and breast milk. While small amounts of the virus have been found in saliva, there have been no known cases of transmission by kissing or other contact with saliva, tears, or sweat. HIV enters the body through its mucous membranes (the lining of the rectum, the walls of the vagina, the inside of the mouth and throat). The virus cannot enter through the skin unless the skin is broken or cut and another person's body fluids enter the bloodstream. The virus also cannot be transmitted through the air by sneezing and coughing. This is why there is absolutely no danger in casual non-body-fluid contact with people who have HIV.

HIV has a long incubation period, which means that a person can have the virus for many years without knowing it and thus can unwittingly infect others. An individual is defined as having AIDS when he or she both tests positive for HIV and displays evidence of serious damage to the immune system, such as pneumonia or another opportunistic infection. No one yet knows what percentage of people infected with HIV may develop AIDS, but at present it is thought that approximately 50 percent of those infected go on to develop AIDS within ten years. On the other hand, some people who have had the virus for at least fourteen years still show no symptoms of AIDS. Since the only reliable way of telling who is infected with the virus is through the antibody test, it is vitally important to understand and practice behavior that reduces the risk of transmission.

The two main vehicles for transmission are sexual intercourse and the sharing of needles with an infected person. While there has been much press about high-risk groups in the past, it is dangerous to allow this to lead you to think that if you are not homosexual or an intravenous drug user, you cannot become infected. A more accurate assessment of the situation is that *HIV does not recognize risk groups.* In Africa, for example, the overwhelming majority of AIDS cases are heterosexual men and women. And in the United States and elsewhere, the virus is more easily passed from a man to a woman than from a woman to a man. Indeed, a small percentage of HIV transmission initially was caused by blood transfusions with blood infected with HIV. (The risk of being infected with HIV via blood transfusions is now very low; in 1985 a test was developed to screen blood for the presence of HIV.)

Of all persons with AIDS, 10 percent are over fifty years of age; 4 percent over seventy. Most of them received HIV through blood transfusions, and epidemiological studies show that those over age sixty infected with HIV progress more rapidly to full-blown AIDS than those who are younger do; these older individuals also have a more severe set of opportunistic infections, possibly due to the combined effect of age and HIV on the production of T cells. (T cells are special cells in the bloodstream which, in a healthy person, attack infections and thus are the building blocks of our immune system. HIV uses these T cells as factories for the production of more HIV, and over time destroys these cells, thus leaving the infected person with an impaired immune system.) To date in the United States 65 percent of AIDS cases involve homosexual or bisexual men, while 20 percent are intravenous (IV) drug users. But these figures are currently changing. Decreasing rates of HIV infection among homosexual men prove that education and safer sex do work. And safer sex needs to be practiced by both men and women of all ages, heterosexual, bisexual, or homosexual.

To have safer sex and decrease your risk of infection, follow these procedures:

• Avoid any unprotected sexual contact that includes the exchange of body fluids (semen, blood, and perhaps saliva).

• Practice sexual monogamy (that is to say, have only one partner whose only partner is you). Unprotected sex (sex without a condom) with multiple partners greatly increases your risk of HIV infection.

• Use latex condoms in every sexual encounter. (If

you have never used a condom before, you may want to send for "The Safer Sex Condom Guide for Men and Women," published by GMHC, listed on the following page). Nonlatex condoms, such as those made of lamb-skin, do not effectively block the transmission of HIV. Also, spermicides and water-based lubricants containing nonoxyl-9 have been shown to kill HIV. However, never trust the use of spermicides alone; *always* use them along with the latex condoms.

• Avoid unprotected oral sex and/or deep oral kissing, since cuts or sores in the mouth can allow the virus to enter the bloodstream. The presence of genital herpes (on either party) triples the risk of HIV infection during sexual relations with an infected partner.

Many centers throughout the country offer information, support, testing, and help for either people with AIDS or those who think they may be at risk. Most city public health clinics now offer free anonymous counseling and testing for HIV. The HIV antibody test can tell if your body has produced antibodies to HIV, so if you test positive, it means that you have been infected with the virus. While there is no cure for AIDS at this point, many treatments are available for those who test positive and these can delay—or even prevent—the onset of such life-threatening infections as PCP, mentioned above. Furthermore, by greatly prolonging the lives of those infected, they allow more time for better treatments to be developed. This is one of the reasons why it is important to be tested if you think you may be at risk. To find out about the testing center nearest you, call the National AIDS Hotline, listed below. Here are some of the best sources of information about various aspects of AIDS:

AIDS EDUCATION AND INFORMATION RESOURCES

National AIDS Clearinghouse
P.O. Box 6003
Rockville, MD 20850
Phone: 1-800-458-5231
　　(Provides information pamphlets and a materials catalog on request)

National AIDS Hotline
Phone: 1-800-342-2437
TDD (for the hearing impaired) 1-800-243-7889
Spanish 1-800-344-7432
　　(Provides educational pamphlets upon request and the names of other AIDS resources near you)

Gay Men's Health Crisis
Publications/Education Department
129 West 20th Street
New York, NY 10011

or Phone Hotline: 212-807-6655
TDD 212-645-7470 (for the hearing impaired)
    (Provides a wide range of services for men,
women, and children affected by HIV and AIDS.
Upon request will send the following pamphlets:
"AIDS Education Resources"; "HIV and AIDS: The
Basics"; "The Safer Sex Condom Guide for Men and
Women"; and "Medical Answers about AIDS")

American Red Cross
AIDS Education Office
1730 E Street, N.W.
Washington, DC 20006
Phone: 202-434-4074
    (Upon request, provides educational information
on HIV and AIDS)

AIDS Action Council
1875 Connecticut Avenue, 5th floor
Washington, DC 20009
Phone: 202-986-1300
    (Provides information on policy and legislative
issues relating to AIDS)

Hispanic AIDS Forum
121 Avenue of the Americas, Suite 505
New York, NY 10013
Phone: 212-966-6662

(Provides information, referrals and counseling to heterosexual, gay, and bisexual members of the Hispanic community) Telephone operators are bilingual.

GENITAL HERPES

Caused by a virus known as herpes simplex 2, genital herpes affects as many as 40 million Americans, and its incidence is increasing, with 300,000 to 500,000 new cases a year for the past few years. Genital herpes is moderately contagious, usually through sexual contact. It is one of the rare sexually transmitted diseases that can also be contracted through sitting unclothed in an infected place, especially in warm, moist environments such as hot tubs and whirlpools (although this is uncommon).

Symptoms appear in the form of itching and small, painful lesions in the genital area four to seven days after sexual contact. Flu-like symptoms may be present as well as general fatigue. These symptoms often disappear temporarily, only to recur. Most people with the active form of the disease have three or four flare-ups a year, each lasting several days to three weeks. The disease is most contagious during this time. Women with the disease may be at greater risk for cervical cancer.

If blisters or lesions do occur, they are treated with a cleansing salt solution. Secondary infections may be treated or avoided by use of oral sulfonamides. Though there is currently neither a cure nor a prevention for genital herpes, an antiviral drug, acyclovir (Zovirax), can prevent flare-ups of the disease; however, the long-term effects of acyclovir are unknown. Flare-ups may recur if the medication is stopped.

GONORRHEA

It is estimated that close to 3 million people in the United States are infected with gonorrhea annually. Men typically show obvious symptoms two to fourteen days after infection, with a tingling sensation in the urethra, and, shortly thereafter, pain during urination and a discharge from the penis. Some men may be asymptomatic for a period of time. In women, the disease is usually asymptomatic for weeks and even months. When symptoms do occur, they are in the form of a vaginal discharge and/or pain on urination, or frequency of urination.

Antibiotics are the usual treatment. Both men and women are asked to refrain from sexual contact until they are cured, and all of those with whom they have had recent sexual contact should be traced and treated as well.

CHLAMYDIA

This may be the most common of all sexually transmitted diseases in the United States. It is often asymptomatic, especially in women. Any onset of unusual vaginal (women) or urethral (men) discharge should be cause for concern. Additional symptoms include pain on urination in men and frequent urination and painful intercourse in women. Anyone experiencing these symptoms should be tested to rule out other sexually transmitted diseases. Once a diagnosis of chlamydia is made, it is easily treated with antibiotics such as tetracycline. If left untreated, chlamydia can cause urethral infections and inflamed testes in men and inflammation of the Fallopian tubes in women.

SYPHILIS

Syphilis is caused by an infectious organism that enters the lymph glands. If untreated, the disease can unfold over a period of years in three stages, the last of which is a fatal infection of the heart, brain, or other organ. Fortunately, nearly all cases are now detected in the primary stage. Lesions (chancres or sores) appear about four weeks after infection, or skin rashes in six to eight weeks. Penicillin is the antibiotic treatment of all three stages. Sexual activity must stop during treatment, and all with whom you have had sexual contact in the preceding three to twelve months should be identified and treated. You need to be retested by your doctor until all traces of the disease have disappeared. A rising incidence of syphilis in recent years is principally associated with drug addiction and AIDS. Nonetheless, it should be of concern to the general population.

HEPATITIS B

Most people don't realize that hepatitis B is a serious virus that is either sexually transmitted or spread through contact with infected blood or other body fluids. It can cause severe liver damage and may result in chronic hepatitis or even death from related illnesses. An estimated 200,000 Americans are infected with hepatitis B each year, and an estimated 5,000 die of complications from the disease. Hepatitis B is the *only* sexually transmitted virus preventable by vaccine. Any person, regardless of age, who is sexually active outside of a strictly monogamous relationship should receive one of the two vaccines now available. See your physician for advice and access to the vaccines.

IN SUMMARY

The early detection and treatment that have been—and essentially still are—the solution for gonorrhea, syphilis, and most recently chlamydia, as well as the vaccines now available to prevent hepatitis B, are inapplicable to diseases such as genital herpes and especially AIDS. The sole protection against these currently incurable diseases is behavior changes that prevent their contraction in the first place. Earlier we outlined recommended sexual behaviors to lessen the risk of exposure to AIDS, especially the avoidance of unprotected intercourse. In the meantime, we must continue with our research to learn how to control this dangerous and deadly public health threat.

IMPOTENCE BASED ON PHYSICAL CAUSES

WHAT IS IMPOTENCE?

We refer here to impotence as erectile dysfunction—that is, the loss of a man's ability to obtain an erection sufficient to achieve or maintain sexual intercourse—and we will use the terms "impotence" and "erection problem" interchangeably. Rarely do men totally lose the capacity for at least *some* degree of erection; however, less than a full erection can interfere with full sexual expression. The severity of the impotence ranges from being incapable of a total erection some of the time to being incapable most or all of the time. Impotence also refers to the inability to sustain an erection even if one is initially able to have one.

It is estimated that anywhere from 10 to 20 million American men suffer from chronic erection problems or impotence, with perhaps 10 million others having partial dysfunction. This is *not* part of the normal physical process of growing older, even though such problems may increase with age, due to physical illness and other causes. If impotence occurs regularly, you should investigate the cause or causes and treat the condition; do not let your physician or anyone else discourage you from seeking help. According to many experts, up to 90 percent of cases can be improved or even reversed with proper diagnosis and treatment. Therefore a man with impotence *must* be examined medically to determine whether or not a physical condition is acting as a partial or complete cause of this impotence.

WHAT PRODUCES AN ERECTION?

The physiology and psychology of getting and maintaining an erection are complicated and are based on reflexes rather than a man's conscious control. Two sets of messages—stimulation of the penis through touch and/ or stimulation of the brain through erotic thoughts triggered by sights, smells, hearing, fantasies, or memories—are sent to nerve centers in the spinal cord. These nerve centers then send messages to the penile blood vessels, causing them to enlarge and fill with blood (engorge), creating an erection. At the same time, the blood is prevented from leaving or leaking out of the penis. Testosterone and chemicals known as neurotransmitters play an important but as yet unclear role. In adolescents and very young men mental stimulation is often enough to produce an erection, but most men in their late forties and thereafter will often find that they need tactile (either manual or oral) stimulation of the penis, in addition to their erotic thoughts, before an erection occurs. One man in his late sixties who spoke to us reported on the success of this route: "For thirty-six years my wife and I enjoyed an active sex life. But then I began to have difficulty getting an erection. My wife felt she was no longer sexually attractive, and I thought I was a failure. We went to a sex counselor, who told us that in addition to our usual patterns of lovemaking, I now needed physical stimulation to get an erection. We started to do this regularly, with my wife stimulating me by hand prior to intercourse. As a result, our sex life has greatly improved. And as an added plus, once my penis is erect, it stays hard much longer."

AT WHAT AGE ARE ERECTION PROBLEMS LIKELY TO OCCUR?

There has been little reliable scientific information concerning the actual experience of impotence as men grow older. Kinsey documented a decline in potency with age up until the age of fifty, but his sample over fifty was too small to draw conclusions from. Duke University and the Gerontology Research Center of the National Institute on Aging in Baltimore have found a general pattern of decline as well, but with much individual variation. Indeed, a significant proportion of men had stable and even rising patterns of sexual activity with age. For our purposes here, it is clear that erection problems do increase with age (due to illness or other causes—but *not* due to physical aging itself); however, such problems are not inevitable, nor are they by any means always permanent.

THE MIND-BODY ISSUE IN IMPOTENCE

It has long been generally (but falsely) accepted that at least 90 percent of impotence in men over sixty was psychologically based, with only about 10 percent physiologically caused. These figures, quoted since the 1920s, can be traced back to the book *Impotence in the Male*, by one of Freud's colleagues, William Stekel. William Masters and Virginia Johnson, the pioneer sex researchers, arrived at the same conclusions in their laboratory studies of older men, and psychotherapists and sex counselors have continued to promulgate these beliefs. The proportion of psychologically based impotence among men forty to sixty has been estimated to be even higher, at 95 percent. However, more effective diagnostic techniques and a growing understanding of the physiology of impotence are starting to change those views. In the last few years, biomedical researchers, using a variety of more sophisticated measurements and advanced techniques, including sleep studies, have begun to suspect that impotence may have a much higher physiological component, perhaps involving 60 to 70 percent or more of all cases of impotence, *regardless* of age. The rates may be even higher for older men, especially those with vascular problems.

As a general rule, if the onset of impotence is sudden and the course is intermittent, the cause is probably psychological, such as recent widowhood. If the onset is slow—over a period of six months to a year—and the course chronic, the cause is much more likely to be physical.

In this book, we have made an artificial division between physically based and psychologically based impotence, simply to facilitate our discussion. In truth the two are usually intermixed, although there is usually a greater emphasis in one direction or another. The psychological aspects of impotence are discussed in later chapters.

MAJOR CAUSES OF PHYSICALLY BASED IMPOTENCE

In a significant number of cases of impotence, a physical illness has probably remained undetected or at least a mixed diagnosis involving physical as well as emotional components has been overlooked. This helps to explain the estimated 60 percent or higher failure rate from using psychotherapy alone to treat potency problems. According to one classification, the major causes of primarily physically based impotence are listed in order of occurrence as follows:

PHYSICAL PROBLEM

Diabetes mellitus

Vascular insufficiency (arteriosclerosis, hypertension, antihypertensive medications [beta blocker agents])

Radical surgery (prostatectomies, colostomies, cystectomies, etc.)

Trauma (spinal cord injuries, pelvic fractures, etc.)

Hypogonadism and other endocrine disorders

Multiple sclerosis

Peyronie's disease (fibrous cavernitis)

Side effects from medications (estrogens, anticholinergic drugs, excessive tranquilizers, antidepressants, antihypertensive agents, opiates, alcohol, etc.)

Under ideal circumstances, the diagnosis of this kind of sexual dysfunction should be multidisciplinary, potentially involving relevant specialists in internal medicine, endocrinology, neurology, urology, radiology, vascular therapy, psychiatry, psychotherapy, and sex therapy. Any evaluation and treatment should take into account your partner as well. To save both time and money, though, make sure that initial treatment efforts focus on adjusting the dosage of any drug you are taking that is associated with impotence or changing to a similar drug without the adverse side effect of impotence. Do not, however, stop taking a medicine you think may be causing the problem without speaking with your physician. You should also not be surprised to find yourself encouraged to undertake changes in your life-style, including improving your diet, quitting smoking, reducing your alcohol consumption, losing weight, and exercising.

And what diagnostic procedures can you expect to undergo? They may require any and/or all of the following:

• A thorough history, including your past sex life, possible psychiatric and psychological contributors to the impotence, review of alcohol and drug use, and past or present illnesses.

• A physical examination.

• A sleep study, which monitors your erections during sleep. A portable home monitor, called a rigiscan, is a simple and inexpensive method of testing for erections. Minimal erections or the absence of erections during sleep strongly suggests, but does not definitely prove, an organic basis for impotence. For information on clinics that conduct such studies, contact the Association of Sleep Disorders Centers, 604 Second Street, S.W., Rochester, MN 55902.

• Testing of the impotence through other methods. This includes visual stimulation, the use of a vibrator, or a papaverine injection alone or in combination with another medication called phentolamine directly into the penis. These penile injections occasionally produce an erection lasting more than an hour in those who are sexually excited *and* physiologically normal. (This can be very effective psychologically, for it demonstrates to an individual with psychological impotence that he *can* have an erection.) Penile blood flow measurements may be useful, as well as glucose tolerance tests to rule diabetes in or out. Indeed, there should be an endocrinological screening to rule out various hormonal dysfunctions such as thyroid, testosterone, and prolactin abnormalities. It should also measure your level of cholesterol, triglycerides, LDL, and HDL.

While pudendal arteriography (injecting a special dye into the main artery that supplies the penis to study blood flow) can accurately assess penile arterial disease, it is quite expensive and physically invasive. You may choose to estimate penile blood flow through certain blood pressure measurements with or without penile injection of papaverine.

TREATMENT FOR IMPOTENCE

Testosterone

Medical treatment for impotence concentrates on treating specific underlying diseases and, occasionally, successful treatment with hormones. At present, male hormone therapy (sex-steroid replacement) remains controversial and experimental. In fact, replacement of the male hormone testosterone has little known permanent beneficial effect on the sexual problems of older men, particularly impotence, unless there is definitely a proven testicular deficiency in the production of male hormones—such as in hypogonadism, which is quite rare. Any benefit from the added testosterone should show up in three to four weeks, but even in those who do appear to respond, the improvement is generally short-lived. The beneficial effects do not tend to be maintained indefinitely except in those with clear-cut hormone deficiencies. There may also be side effects, such as fluid retention, and evidence indicates that the testosterone may stimulate already existing prostatic growth; thus it should not be given if the prostate gland is enlarged.

Self-Injection/Pharmacotherapy

If you are able to be comfortable with it, the self-injection of vasoactive compounds (called intracavernous pharmacotherapy) directly into the corpora cavernosa (the shaft) of the penis can be valuable in helping produce an erection. In such a treatment you must follow strict sterile procedures, and there should be long-term follow-up.

In the past the most popular substance for this kind of self-injection was a mixture of papaverine hydrochloride and phentolamine. However, the U.S. Food and Drug Administration has not officially approved using papaverine for this purpose, and its manufacturer, Eli Lilly, states that the drug "is not indicated for the treatment of impotence by intracorporeal injection." Nonetheless, many urologists use it for this purpose, and the American Urological Association recognizes its value. Patients who have mild to moderate vascular-based impotence are usually the best candidates for this type of treatment. (Ordinarily, self-injection therapy is not effective in the presence of severe vascular disease.) Prostaglandin–E-1 (PGE-1), another drug that can be injected directly into the penis—has now been found to be effective in many patients, even those who do not respond to papaverine. Due to its few side effects, many urologists are currently using this drug alone or in combination with papaverine or phentolamine or both.

Long-term injection therapy can eventually prove to be a problem, particularly when it comes to high doses of papaverine. The quality of the erections produced sometimes declines over time. And occasionally, priapism—sustained erection lasting longer than four hours—can occur. (If these prolonged erections last more than four hours, they must be reversed. This can be done either by aspiration of a small amount of blood or by injecting dilute epinephrine or phenylephrine.) Lastly, there can be intense scarring of the penis, which may make implantation of a prosthesis, if it is needed later, difficult or even impossible.

In spite of all these difficulties, many find the self-injections invaluable and become quite accustomed to them, just as diabetics become used to insulin injections. Self-injection works best in those whose impotence is caused by nerve damage (as a result of spinal cord injury, lumbar disc disease, radical pelvic surgery, multiple sclerosis, or juvenile onset diabetes) and in those affected by poor circulation. However, some hypertensive individuals experienced prolonged erections as a side effect of injecting combined papaverine hydrochloride and phentolamine mesylate into the penis. Men who experience psychogenic impotence can also use the self-injection method temporarily.

External Vacuum Devices

Other men use external vacuum devices (EVDs) to obtain and maintain erections. For this procedure, you fit a plastic-cylinder vacuum device over the limp penis, attach a piece of plastic tubing to an opening in the end of the device, and then suck the air out with a syringe, a pump, or your mouth. (Battery-driven devices are also available.) This produces a gentle vacuum that encourages blood flow into the penis, creating an erection. Once a full erection occurs, a wide rubber band, or constriction ring (they are available in different sizes), stored on the end of the cylinder nearest the base of the penis, is slipped around the penis's base to retain the blood, thus maintaining the erection. According to Dr. E. Douglas Whitehead, a urologist and director of the

Association for Male Sexual Dysfunction in New York City, EVDs have proven to be up to 80 percent successful in creating and maintaining an erection sufficient for the duration of intercourse. So, compared to an implant, this method is much less expensive, and does not permanently alter the penis since no surgery is involved.

You do need a physician's prescription to obtain an EVD. And bear in mind that its long-term safety and effectiveness are still being evaluated. Men on anticoagulant therapy or those who have blood abnormalities should not use EVDs. Also, a small proportion of men report that their ejaculation is blocked and this may result in pain. But in general, most find that an orgasm is both possible and pleasurable, and that their partner's satisfaction is also high, especially when their relationship is otherwise supportive. If you wish more information on these devices and/or have other questions on male sexual dysfunction, contact the Association for Male Sexual Dysfunction, 520 East 72nd Street, New York, NY 10021, or phone 212-794-1616.

Another external vacuum device, the Synergist Erection System, consists of a condom-like semi-rigid sheath of silicone. It also uses suction to create a vacuum and achieve an erection, but unlike the cylinder described earlier, it can be left on as long as the user wishes.

Dietary Changes

Although it is rare, a zinc deficiency in the daily diet may interfere with your normal hormone production and thereby affect your sexual functioning. To circumvent this, obtain zinc by eating shellfish, seafood, meats, and certain whole grains, nuts, and legumes, or in multiple vitamins.

Implants

Penile prostheses or implants have been rather widely used to treat impotence. However, they have fallen out of favor as a first-line treatment because of surgical complications and mechanical malfunction. As of 1992, some 250,000 to 300,000 men in the United States have had both inflatable and noninflatable prostheses of various types implanted, and in March of the same year the FDA announced it would start evaluating the safety of these implants as medical devices. These implants have been used to treat permanent organic impotence, especially when it is due to diabetes or vascular problems, and in a few instances, psychological impotence that has not responded to psychotherapy. Such devices do not interfere with the pleasurable feelings of intercourse as long as a man's nerves of sensation in the genital area are in working order. While the implants themselves do not produce a climax or increase sexual desire, those men who could have an orgasm before the surgery can do so afterward. The three main manufacturers of prostheses are American Medical Systems of Minnetonka, Minnesota, Mentor Corporation of Santa Barbara, California, and Dacomed of Minneapolis. They will provide information about their products in response to letters and calls.

In order to reach a decision about the desirability of a penile implant you should know that the following are not considered good candidates for penile prosthesis:

• Men with untreated acute and severe depression. The depression should be successfully treated first.

• Those with serious psychosis or brain disease.

• Men with severe personality disorders, including the chronically dissatisfied.

• Those with severe and complicated marital problems.

• Men whose impotence is not clearly organic.

• Men who have health conditions that contraindicate elective surgery.

It is more advisable to consider a penile implant when:

• It is clear that the impotence is primarily a chronic organic problem (caused, for example, by diabetes or vascular disease or by problems associated with rectal or prostate surgery, pelvic nerve injury, or spinal cord injury).

• External devices do not work, and penile injections are not an option, or have failed.

• Sexual desire is strong and both you and your partner greatly value intercourse.

• You engage in sexual activity with your partner even in the absence of actual intercourse.

• The presence of impotence per se is having a destructive effect on your relationship.

• As a couple you have a realistic understanding of what may be achieved, and both of you approve of the surgery.

It is ideal if both you and your partner are involved in pre- and post-surgical consultation. Moreover, sex counseling in addition to the surgery is essential, since couples often need explicit instructions on how best to use a prosthesis.

What are the risks you encounter from such implants as these? There is always danger of infection at the time of insertion, as well as the possibility of mechanical malfunction. Current estimates of as high as 90 percent surgical success are likely exaggerated or, at the very least, based on unreliable data. In addition, satisfaction with a prosthesis may very well decline over time. The inflatable devices are reported to have a higher rate of failure and earlier prostheses often required another operation. Most such failures involve leaks from various parts of the apparatus, including saline leaks from the inflatable tubes.

Some believe that in general, implants are *not* considered to be lifetime devices, and will eventually need to be removed or replaced. Nonetheless, many urologists have a positive attitude about them, stating that current implants show vast improvements over earlier versions. The 1993 National Institutes of Health Consensus Conference on Impotence echoed this optimism, generally agreeing that implants represent an important treatment option for chronic impotence. The U.S. Food and Drug Administration has begun requiring better monitoring of success rates on the part of doctors and better disclosure of problems by implant manufacturers.

Revascularization

Arteriosclerosis and conditions such as peripheral vascular disease, sickle cell anemia, traumas or accidents to the penis and surrounding area, or simply an insufficient blood flow to the penis since birth can affect the circulation of blood to the penis. Revascularization, or surgery involving the shifting of blood vessels, is used to restore normal blood circulation to the penis. While this kind of surgery is still evolving, and results are currently disappointing, it shows promise for the future. However, revascularization is almost never recommended for diabetic impotence. Some surgeons feel revascularization is not indicated in cases of advanced general arteriosclerosis. Others believe that arteriosclerosis often advances segmentally, and if it is more advanced in the penis than in other parts of the body, revascularization in that area may result in many more years of functioning. In one vascular condition, Leriche's syndrome, there is an intermittent reduction of the penile blood supply needed for erection. Aching, fatigue, weakness, cramping, numbness, discomfort in the thigh, pain in the calf, or limping may accompany this syndrome. Rest relieves many of the symptoms, and surgery can eliminate the limp and restore sexual potency.

Questionable Treatments for Impotence

Because impotence is such a widespread concern, a host of questionable treatments have evolved. Folklore is full of reputed "remedies." Doctors have been known to prescribe oysters, greens, and massive amounts of vitamins B_{12} and E. There are also "youth doctors" and nonmedical entrepreneurs who produce and sell countless substances and gadgets advertised to rejuvenate sexual potency. Older people are often the targets of fraudulent consumer schemes and devices that promise to "make you look younger" and "guarantee" to prevent or cure impotence. The U.S. Postal Service, which brings action against those engaged in obtaining money or property through the mails by means of false representations, provided us with a representative list of worthless nostrums and alleged aphrodisiacs. Among the popular names are "Mexican Spanish Fly in Liquid Form," "Instant Love Potion," "Sex Stimulant for Women," "Mad Dog Weed," "Magic Lure," "Super Nature Tablets," "European Love Drops," "Linga Pendulum Penis Enlarger and Strengthener," "Big Ox," made of vitamins and minerals, and VBE-21, advertised as the "Doctor's Pill for Loss of Sex Drive." On page 106 we list by popular and scientific names a variety of alleged aphrodisiacs. *Watch out for them.* If they seem to work, it is only through the power of suggestion, and any "cure" is likely to be temporary. Some are extremely dangerous. Spanish fly, for example, will not improve erections, yet some men continue to hope that it will work. An older man wrote us: "I wish you could tell me where I can get a small amount of Spanish fly. I will be careful with it as I am seventy-one and wouldn't want anything to go wrong." Our reply was to let him know that Spanish fly was not effective in improving erections and could possibly lead to death! Even small doses may produce kidney failure and shock within twenty-four hours.

The Food and Drug Administration (FDA) began an attempt to ban the sale of all nonprescription aphrodisiacs in mid-1985. The ban does not, however, cover products such as ginseng that do not claim to be aphrodisiacs but nevertheless have that association in the public mind. Chinese ginseng, readily available in health food stores, is used in the belief that it preserves health, increases alertness, and improves endurance. Its aphrodisiac action has been interpreted (but not scientifically proven) as a consequence of improved health, which produces a return to normal sexual desire and functioning. Taken in moderation, ginseng has no known adverse side effects.

One aphrodisiac that may at least partially live up

to its reputation and, after studies, eventually graduate
to the role of a proven drug is yohimbine, an extract

SOME FALSE APHRODISIACS

Alcohol	Especially wines
Cantharidin	Tincture of *Cantharis vesicatoria* (Spanish fly)
Capsicum	Extract of *Capsicum frutescens* (cayenne pepper from South America)
Cimicifugin	Resin from *Cimicifuga racemosa* (black snakeroot)
Cubeb	Oleoresin from *Piper cubeba* (from Java)
Damiana	From leaves of *Turnera diffusa* (from Mexico)
Ergot	Alkaloids from *Claviceps purpurea*
Marijuana	*Cannabis sativa*
Nux vomica	Extract from seeds of *Strychnos nux-vomica*
Sanguinaria	Extract from *Sanguinaria canadensis* (bloodroot)
Vitamin E	d-alpha-tocopherol

from the bark of the African yohimbe tree. Yohimbine,
an alpha blocker, induces dilation of certain blood vessels in the penis. Thus far it has been found to be mod-
estly useful, if given in high dosages, in treating

organically based erectile dysfunction. But reports do indicate that it may trigger panic attack in men who are severely anxious. Its other possible side effects include sweating, nausea, and changes in blood pressure.

In 1992 came support for the hypothesis that nitric oxide is involved in smooth muscle relaxation in the corpora cavernosa, thus making penile erection possible. This new understanding of the mechanism of tumescence may lead to new treatments—and possibly the development of a removable patch of nitric oxide, which could be placed on the penis itself in order to keep the penis engorged and erect.

IN SUMMARY

In 1993, it was estimated that more than a million men were currently receiving treatment for impotence in the United States: A million received pharmacotherapy (or self-injections), 30,000 vacuum systems, 20,000 penile implants, and 1,500 vascular surgical repair.

And recently the diagnosis and treatment of impotence has received unprecedented attention in the media and medical community. There has been a rapid increase in the number of information and counseling centers set up throughout the country. Many of these centers and self-help groups have been formed by sufferers of impotence, so that individuals and couples can receive medical and psychological support from both health professionals and fellow impotence sufferers. The atmosphere at these self-help meetings is structured to be open, honest, and emotionally supportive. Read on for specific sources of information or counseling:

Impotents Anonymous, Suite 292, 2020 Pennsylvania Ave. NW, Washington, D.C., 20006. For counseling and support, individuals and couples can contact Impotents Anonymous (IA), for impotent men, or I-ANON, for the partners of impotent men. Founded in 1983, this non-profit organization has over a hundred chapters throughout the United States and provides anonymous counseling and support. The organization also has audio- and videotapes on impotence, and offers a list of health-care professionals in your area who specialize in impotence. A free brochure, "Answers to the Most Often-Asked Questions About Impotence," is available by calling 1-800-669-1603.

Recovery of Male Impotence (ROMP) (For a brochure that describes some of the causes and treatments for impotence, as well as a list of ROMP chapters nationwide, write to ROMP Center, 27211 Lahser Road, Suite 208, Southfield, Michigan 48034, or call 1-800-TEL-ROMP.) ROMP has programs in twenty-seven hospitals in ten states to diagnose and treat impotence. ROMP groups, which meet on a regular basis, provide support to men who are beginning to deal with the problem and also welcome those who have already been treated for impotence to share their experiences. During meetings, health-care professionals discuss topics such as symptoms, testing, treatments, and the emotional impact of impotence. Partners of impotent men are welcome.

The Association for Male Sexual Dysfunction, 520 East 72nd Street, New York, New York 10021, 212-794-1616, is a multispecialty group of physicians that offers evaluation, diagnosis, and treatment of male sexual dysfunctions. The specialties covered include internal medicine, endocrinology, diagnostic radiology, neurophysiological testing, urology, neurology, sex therapy, psychiatry, vascular surgery and sleep consultation.

Impotence Information Center, Department USA, P.O. Box 9, Minneapolis, Minnesota 55440, 1-800-843-4315, is run by a maker of penile prostheses. A free booklet, *Impotence Help in the USA*, is available.

American Association of Sex Educators, Counselors and Therapists (ASSECT), 435 North Michigan Avenue, Suite 1717, Chicago, Illinois 60611-4067, provides a list of its members in your state if you send a business-size self-addressed stamped envelope (SASE).

American Foundation for Urologic Disease, Inc., 300 West Pratt Street, Suite 401, Baltimore, Maryland 21201, 410-727-2908, provides information and will answer questions on Peyronie's disease, prostate disease, impotence, incontinence, and other urological disorders. You may either write or phone.

CHAPTER 4

❧ ❧

THE EFFECTS OF
DRUGS (INCLUDING
ALCOHOL) AND SURGERY
ON YOUR SEXUALITY

DRUGS

Drugs—prescription or otherwise—can and do cause serious sexual problems for both men and women. Their impact on sexuality may be major or subtle. Doctors often fail to consider the sexual consequences of drugs they prescribe, and those who take them are often unaware that their medications may influence their sexual desire and/or functioning.

If you are having sexual problems, then it would be wise to consider whether the drugs you are using are having a negative impact on your sexuality. A study reported in 1983 in the *Journal of the American Medical Association* found that *25 percent* of sexual problems in men were either caused or complicated by medications. Less is known about the effects of drugs on female sexuality—but the assumption is that those drugs that affect men will affect women as well. Some drugs interfere with the autonomic nervous system, which is involved in normal sexual response, while others affect mood and alertness or change the production or action of sex hormones. Read on for more detailed information.

PRESCRIPTION DRUGS

Tranquilizers, antidepressants, and certain antihypertensives (agents for controlling high blood pressure) have all been implicated in impaired erection in men. Their effects on women are less understood, largely because in the past, women were often not included in drug trials.

Tranquilizers

Strong tranquilizers such as Mellaril (thioridazine) and other phenothiazines may cause failure to obtain an erection or to ejaculate even when the capacity for erection remains. Any tranquilizing drug—even a mild one such as Librium (chlordiazepoxide)—can also act as a depressant on both male and female sexual feelings.

Antidepressants

Antidepressants such as imipramine hydrochloride (Tofranil) may inhibit sexual desire. According to two reports in the February 1985 *Journal of Clinical Psychopharmacology*, adverse sexual side effects have been reported with all standard antidepressants. However, you must weigh the impact of the side effects against your need for the antidepressant, and act accordingly. And remember: not everyone necessarily experiences the side effects in the first place.

Antihypertensives

Antihypertensive medications are the most common cause of impaired erection. Blocking agents, one class of antihypertensive drugs, include methyldopa (Aldomet), which reduces the flow of blood into the pelvic area and so inhibits erection.

Thomas, sixty-two, had always believed himself to be in good health, and so was surprised when his physician told him he had high blood pressure. The doctor recommended changes in his diet, as well as an exercise program. Thomas's blood pressure improved somewhat, but still ran about 130 over 95. The doctor thought it important that Thomas be on antihypertensive medication, and put him on methyldopa. Thomas's blood pressure was soon under control, but as a consequence of the drug, he was often unable to have an erection. He discussed this with his physician, and once an ACE inhibitor (see below), a class of antihypertensive agents that appear to have fewer adverse effects on sexuality, was substituted for methyldopa, Thomas's erection problems disappeared. (Sometimes efforts to vary or lower the dosage of antihypertensive medications are not always so successful; however, in Thomas's case, things worked out well.)

Another drug used against hypertension, guanethidine (Ismelin), may inhibit ejaculation by blocking the nerves involved. Up to two-thirds of men taking this medication have reported problems. Guanethidine can also cause retrograde ejaculation (see page 137). The common antihypertensive reserpine can decrease sexual interest or, at times, induce impotence. Even the diuretics given for high blood pressure can cause problems, as Bob, age sixty-eight, found out when he was placed on a diuretic for this very problem. When he found that he was unable to have an erection, it never occurred to him that the diuretic might be responsible. He attributed his changing status to aging. Fortunately, his physician asked him if there were any side effects from the medication, specifically in terms of his erectile function. When the doctor learned of Bob's problem, he lowered the dosage of the medication and Bob soon reported returning to normal.

Those antihypertensive drugs that are frequently implicated in impaired sexuality include those with peripheral and central actions of sympatholytic or beta-adrenergic blocking activity. Calcium channel blockers, angiotensin-converting enzyme (ACE) inhibitors, and peripheral vasodilators do *not* cause significant sexual dysfunction.

If you develop sexual problems after taking antihypertensive medications, *do not* discontinue or decrease your medications without telling your doctor. Doing so would be very dangerous, as your medications could be preventing a stroke.

Your doctor may be able to help solve your sexual problems without endangering your health. Some alternatives are to switch antihypertensives, to use only a diuretic, and/or to reduce dosages when feasible. In fact, many physicians no longer prescribe medications for mild to moderate hypertension until their patients have first tried to bring their blood pressure under control by lowering salt intake and by exercise and weight reduction. When drugs *are* necessary, one study suggests that one of the most effective regimens—with the least likelihood of sexual impairment—is a combination of an oral diuretic, hydralazine, and propranolol. However, propranolol, promoted at first for its lack of sexual side effects, has now been implicated as affecting sexuality, especially when higher dosages are used.

Other Drugs

What other drugs should you be concerned about? The corticosteroids taken for arthritis may produce at least temporary impotence. Analgesics (pain medications) may reduce sensitivity and therefore affect male sexual capacity. Cimetidine (Tagamet), used in the treatment of duodenal ulcers and one of the most widely sold medicines in the United States, can cause impotence. One possible substitute for cimetidine that should not impair your sexuality is ranitidine (Zantac).

ALCOHOL

You should be aware that alcohol is also a drug. Pharmacologically it is a depressant rather than a stimulant, though in small amounts it may relax sexual inhibition in a pleasant manner. In larger amounts, however, it usually interferes with sexual performance, reducing potency in males and arousal and orgasmic ability in both sexes. At the very least, alcohol often produces drowsiness, which then interferes with sex. The excessive use of alcohol is a frequent and too-little-recognized factor in sexual problems, and often those who abuse alcohol fail to realize how much they are actually drinking.

Certainly, most people would never have realized that Mary, age sixty-five, had a drinking problem. Mary herself never suspected it. Over the years, especially since her husband's death, she had begun drinking more frequently. Rather than one or two drinks a day, she now regularly had at least three or four. Since her husband's death, various men had expressed interest in her, but Mary had lost all sexual desire. She considered this a kind of loyalty to her husband. During her annual visit to her doctor, he asked about her alcohol intake and began to suspect alcohol abuse. Mary denied having a problem. But one day she had a serious fall on the stairs that even she could see had been related to her drinking. Her doctor strongly recommended that she go to the Hazelton alcohol treatment center in Minnesota for treatment. She took his advice and some months later, was recovering and doing quite well. Moreover, she was surprised to find that her sexual feelings and desires had returned.

How does alcohol intake affect the members of both sexes? For men, even a few drinks before sex can impair sexual performance. Erections may be less firm and ejaculation more difficult. But though this effect is temporary and reversible in terms of physical capacity, it can frighten a man into believing he is impotent, and the fear itself may then prolong the impotence.

Up to 80 percent of men who drink heavily are believed to suffer serious sexual side effects, including impotence, sterility, or loss of sexual desire. Many of the effects of moderate to heavy drinking may be reversible if the drinking stops in time. However, heavy drinking over a long period irreversibly destroys testicular cells, leaving men with shrunken testicles. Both sexual drive and sexual capacity can be damaged. Hormone production is often affected, resulting in a decrease in testosterone and a drop in the sperm count. Total sterility as well as impotence result. Chronic heavy drinking can also produce liver and brain damage that leads to an excess production of female hormones and a feminized body appearance.

Women are affected by alcohol in many of the same ways as men. More than one drink before a sexual encounter can interfere with arousal and the ability to reach orgasm. Chronic heavy use of alcohol in the middle years can damage the ovaries, causing menstrual and ovulatory abnormalities and a decrease in estrogen production. This in turn may lead to early menopause and signs of premature aging. Atrophy of the breasts, uterus, and vaginal walls and lessened lubrication in the vagina are common.

One's tolerance for alcohol decreases with age (one cause is changing kidney excretory power), so that smaller and smaller amounts may begin to produce negative effects. It is wise to avoid drinking altogether for several hours before a sexual encounter, or at least to limit alcohol intake to one drink. If you choose to drink regularly, limit yourself to a maximum of one and a half ounces of hard liquor, one six-ounce glass of wine, or two eight-ounce glasses of beer in any twenty-four-hour period. Remember, too, that alcohol is very dangerous in combination with narcotic and non-narcotic drugs such as sleeping pills, sedatives, painkillers, antihistamines, antidepressants, and tranquilizers, because it can pyramid their effects. So *if you are taking drugs, do not drink without first discussing it with your doctor.*

TOBACCO

Because of its nicotine content, tobacco is also a drug, although it is not usually categorized as one. It, too, may factor in impotence. There is an old German saying about male erectile capacity: *"Rauchen macht schlump"*—"Smoking makes [it] dangle." Toxic changes in the blood from nicotine may affect sex hormones. There is some evidence that men who smoke have lower levels of testosterone. Nicotine also constricts blood vessels, in some cases enough to affect blood flow to the penis. Long-term smokers with athero-sclerosis or peripheral vascular disease can become impotent. It is suspected that smoking has effects on female sexuality as well, but studies have not yet been done in this area.

NARCOTICS AND OTHER DRUGS

Regular users of opiates like morphine and heroin are often sexually impaired. Males who are addicted are usually impotent.

While cocaine initially heightens sexual sensation in both sexes as a result of euphoria, increased energy, and heightened self-confidence, with its habitual use individuals experience a lowered sense of self-esteem, together with insomnia, fatigue, anxiety, depression, and even paranoia, hallucinations, and seizures. Women become nonorgasmic and men impotent. A national telephone aid line—800-COCAINE (that is, 1-800-262-2463)—has been established for those who want help in stopping cocaine use.

Marijuana can lead to decreased sexual interest and impotence as well as the drying out of the mucous membranes in the sex organs. Amphetamines can produce impotence, delayed or no ejaculation in men, and inhibition of orgasms in women. Regular users of such barbiturates as sedatives and hypnotics (sleeping pills) may become impotent.

A rare but exceedingly destructive condition called priapism can occur in men who use certain drugs such as butyl (or isobutyl) nitrate, known also as poppers, to stimulate more frequent and longer-lasting erections. An antidepressant drug, trazodone (Desyrel), can also cause similar problems. Priapism is a persistent and often painful erection of the penis caused by blood becoming trapped in the corpora cavernosa—the chambers in the penis that fill with blood to create erections. The erection does not subside on its own, and emergency medical care is needed within twenty-four hours or less to avoid permanent damage to the penis and almost certain permanent impotence. Partial priapism—any unusual period of persistent erection that eventually goes away by itself—is a sign that something is wrong; seek medical advice and treatment.

AVOIDING PROBLEMS

Health-care professionals who prescribe or monitor the use of drugs should be thoroughly familiar with each drug's potential for adverse effects on sexuality. (Dr. James W. Long's annually updated book *The Essential Guide to Prescription Drugs* [HarperCollins] is a useful reference, as is Kathryn Watterson's *The Safe Medicine Book* [Ivy Books, 1988].) It is important that doctors obtain their patient's sexual history before giving any drug that may affect sexuality. This allows comparisons to be made before and after drugs are taken. Physicians should review their patient's drug usage regularly, including their use of prescription and other over-the-counter drugs, alcohol, and tobacco. Plus, doctors should carefully explain the potential side effects of drugs to their patients.

Most drug-caused sexual impairment is reversible if the responsible drug is reduced, removed, or replaced by another. (Impairment due to chronic alcoholism and possibly marijuana use may *not* be reversible.) In cases of serious illness, sexuality may have to be partially—or even totally—sacrificed for a period of time in order to obtain the beneficial effects of drugs that are essential to treatment. But in many cases, alternative drugs, lower dosages, or other treatment altogether can be given. For example, an antihypertensive drug that may adversely affect one person's sexuality will not affect another's. Weigh the possible sexual side effects of a drug against the risks of a disease; your—the patient's—preference should be a crucial factor in the resulting decision.

SURGERY

It's certainly not surprising that most people are apprehensive about any and all surgery on their sex organs. In addition to the usual risks involved in any surgical procedure, they are dreading possible sexual consequences. Many women mistakenly believe removal of the womb (hysterectomy) or of a breast (mastectomy) makes them "less of a woman." And men worry that prostate surgery means the end of sex life altogether. It is reassuring to know that the medical evidence does not support many of these fears, as long as the surgeons are skilled, knowledgeable about the possible problems, and sensitive to their patients' interest in preserving sexual functioning.

HYSTERECTOMY

A hysterectomy is the removal of the womb or uterus. In addition, the ovaries and Fallopian tubes may also be removed (this is called bilateral salpingo-ovariectomy). It is estimated that more than half of all women will have had a hysterectomy by age sixty-five, making this the most common major operation performed in the United

States. However, the evidence is growing that a proportion of these operations—such as those performed to remove the ovaries and uterus as a preventative against future cancers in these organs—is unnecessary. The slim risk of contracting cancer must be weighed against the many benefits of avoiding such surgeries. So if you are considering a hysterectomy, we strongly suggest that you receive a second, or even a third, opinion. HERS (Hysterectomy Educational Resources and Services) offers free phone counseling and support to women and their families faced with the question of surgery. Their quarterly newsletter is available at $20 per year. Write 422 Bryn Mawr Avenue, Bala Cynwyd, Pennsylvania 19004.

Many hysterectomies are done because of the presence of benign (noncancerous) tumors called fibroids, which are not troublesome so long as they remain small but may require surgery if they enlarge, cause bleeding, or involve other organs. Prolapse of the uterus ("fallen uterus"); cancer of the cervix, the endometrium (lining of the uterus), or related organs; and severe, uncontrollable infection or bleeding are other legitimate reasons for a hysterectomy.

It is often said there is no medical evidence that careful removal of the uterus causes impairment of sexual sensations. Yet some women greatly depend on sensations from the cervix and womb to achieve orgasm through deep penile penetration; after hysterectomy they must learn other methods of arousal, such as more focus on clitoral stimulation. The rhythmic contractions of the uterus during orgasm are, of course, gone as a result of a hysterectomy. During the surgical repair, surgeons should be careful to avoid shortening the vagina, which can lead to problems with intercourse. Correct positioning of the wound repair in the back of the vagina is also important. If intercourse is resumed too early after hysterectomy, there can be pain due to incomplete healing in the vagina. Most physicians recommend waiting six to eight weeks before sexual activity is begun again.

Many surgeons and women themselves warn that a period of emotional instability commonly begins about the third or fourth day after a hysterectomy and lasts two to five or ten days or longer. Depression, sleep disturbances, fatigue, listlessness, weight gain, loss of appetite, weeping, and irritability may occur—they are physical and/or emotional responses to the surgery. If symptoms are severe or long lasting, they may require psychotherapeutic, hormonal, or other intentions. Most women regain their equilibrium naturally, although many claim that it takes six months or longer to fully recover physically, especially if the ovaries have been removed. *How to Avoid a Hysterectomy* by Lynn Payer (Pantheon Books, 1987) and *Hysterectomy: Before and After* by Winnifred B. Cutler (HarperCollins, 1988) are useful guides for dealing with the issues surrounding hysterectomy.

Removal of all or parts of a woman's childbearing

apparatus, powerful symbols of womanhood, often does have significant psychological effects. If the woman sees the surgery as symbolic "castration," she needs to resolve this, either on her own or with outside help. She must understand that removal of the sexual organs need not eradicate sexuality, cause her to feel unattractive, or diminish her womanliness. Short-term preoperative and postoperative counseling, ideally with her partner present, can do much to allay a woman's fears and misapprehensions. Group discussions with other women who have had hysterectomies can be especially helpful; women's health centers or hospital social workers may be able to arrange this.

Hysterectomies *can* have positive effects on sexuality, particularly if they are done to relieve painful or debilitating conditions like infection, urinary incontinence, heavy bleeding, or endometriosis. A return to pain-free good health can be a potent aphrodisiac!

MASTECTOMY

While most breast lumps (80 to 90 percent) are found to be benign upon biopsy, unfortunately the likelihood of breast cancer increases with age. Full or partial breast removal, or mastectomy, is performed when a lump in the breast is found to be malignant (cancerous).

In spite of current controversy over whether breast cancer begins in the breast or is a systemic disease beginning elsewhere, most physicians emphasize the early detection of lumps as a major means of combating the disease. In addition to routine examination by your physician and the use of newer techniques to help him or her in diagnosis (for example, mammography by low-voltage X rays), you should definitely undertake regular monthly self-examinations. For information on breast cancer, call the cancer hotline at the National Cancer Institute, Bethesda, MD 20003, 1-800-422-6237. We also recommend Linda Dackman's *Upfront, Sex and the Post-Mastectomy Woman* (Viking, 1990) and *Dr. Susan Love's Breast Book* by Dr. Susan Love and Karen Lindsay (Addison Wesley, 1990).

There are different kinds of mastectomy, ranging from removal of the lump(s) and some adjacent tissue only to the removal of the entire breast, the surrounding lymph glands, and chest muscles. These operations have understandable psychological implications for many women, because they not only change the outward appearance of the body but visibly alter a specific symbol of sexuality. Periodic depression, with its subsequent consequences for one's sex life, is common and expected during the first year or two after a mastectomy. Aesthetic reactions to breast removal can be more difficult than with a hysterectomy, which leaves no obvious signs beyond an abdominal scar.

Although there is no physiological change in sexual capacity after mastectomy, women may temporarily lose their sexual desire out of embarrassment, inability to accept the loss of the breast, and fear that they have become less attractive to their sexual partners. They are also afraid the absence of the breast will be noticeable in public. Some women choose breast reconstruction, using either silicone or saline implants or tissue from elsewhere in the body. However, in 1992 the FDA ordered sharp reductions in the use of silicone gel breast implants until extensive studies of their safety can be carried out. Saline implants are also under study. (For up-to-date information on implants, call the National Cancer Institute at 1-800-422-6237.) To immediately relieve anxiety about their public appearance, women can choose to wear a properly fitting prosthetic bra. However, reactions to breast loss by the women themselves and their partners are not always so easily resolved.

One useful technique is to talk frankly with other women who have already experienced a breast loss. Some physicians and hospitals arrange for such volunteers to counsel women prior to and following surgery. The Reach to Recovery program of the American Cancer Society, begun by Terese Lazar in 1952, is a rehabilitation program for women who have had breast surgery. (A helpful free booklet, "Reach to Recovery," is available from local units of the American Cancer Society.) The program is designed to help with physical, psychological, and cosmetic concerns, and utilizes a carefully selected and trained corps of volunteers who have adjusted successfully to their own surgery. Other forms of

individual and group support can be immensely reliev-
ing as well.

Men, too, need a period of adjustment to work out
their feelings about breast surgery in their partners. In
some cities, Reach to Recovery uses male volunteers to
help men adjust to their wives' mastectomies, while The
Cancer Care Foundation has support groups for cancer
patients' "significant others." In strong relationships,
time and affection often take care of any disturbed feelings following the removal of a breast.

When Hannah, age sixty, received a phone call
from her physician telling her that her mammogram
looked suspicious, she hurried in to be examined. A
small lump was found. She and her husband were hop-
ing, of course, that it would be benign at biopsy. Unfortunately, that was not the case; she had cancer. After
exploring various possibilities, Hannah had a mastectomy of her left breast. She was given a good chance of
recovery because the cancer had been found early. But
Hannah was anxious about her appearance. At first she
would not let her husband see or touch her scar; however, he wisely insisted. Now she says, "I had more
trouble dealing with it than my husband." Both report
that they have become comfortable and feel even more
tender toward one another than before the operation.

However, severe and prolonged emotional upset
may require professional psychotherapy. Do not avoid
seeking aid in such cases; the odds are that it will help

greatly, whether the problem lies with you or with your mate.

To speed up the resumption of a normal sex life after a mastectomy, you should practice the following:

• Involve your partner in all aspects of the discussions around a mastectomy.

• Have your partner see the surgical repair as early as possible after surgery, so the process of adjustment can begin.

• Resume sexual activity as soon as possible.

• Find comfortable sexual positions. For the first weeks and months, your surgical repair will be sensitive. A preferred sexual position is to have your partner on top, supporting his upper body with his arms. This leaves you in a relaxed position on your back, with no stress on your chest area.

• Decide together whether you want to wear a prosthesis (a padded bra) during sexual contact or whether you, as a couple, can be comfortable without it. Many couples eventually eliminate the need for the cover-up.

• Share feelings openly and support each other emotionally. Both of you are likely to have periods of depression and anxiety due to the fear of death that cancer brings and to the loss of a valued body part. Those who can share such feelings may not need further counseling after the initial adjustment period.

Today breast cancer treatment is highly controversial. A few years ago most surgeons performed what is called the Halsted radical mastectomy. It involved removing the entire breast, underlying muscles, and the nearby lymph nodes, thereby leaving a woman with a sunken chest wall and impaired mobility of the arm. When it was discovered that surgeons in countries such as Canada and England were removing much less breast tissue and getting nearly identical survival rates, American surgeons began changing their approach. Many now perform either a modified radical mastectomy, which removes less muscle and fewer lymph nodes, or lumpectomies, which remove only the lump itself. These surgeries have been found to be equally as effective as the more radical procedures. Radiation therapy may be used as well.

Drug therapies, also called adjuvant therapy, are an additional treatment that cancer specialists are beginning to use, along with the surgery, to improve survival chances. Tamoxifen, an artificial hormone that blocks estrogen, has recently shown promise. Chemotherapy—drugs that attack cancer cells—is also used.

VAGINAL RECONSTRUCTION

Women who have had a number of children, difficult childbirths, or tears in the opening of the vagina at the time of childbirth may have an excessively enlarged vagina. Anterior and posterior plastic repair, a surgical procedure, may reconstruct the vagina effectively and make sex more pleasurable. This is a delicate operation and requires an especially skilled surgeon who is also sensitive to the woman's needs. We recommend a second medical opinion on the advisability of this surgery.

PROSTATECTOMY

Prostatectomy involves surgical removal of part or all of the prostate, a gland located at the base of the urethra. As men grow older, up to half of them experience significant enlargement of the prostate. This usually begins after age forty or fifty, and almost all men over fifty have some degree of enlargement. Fifty to 75 percent have noticeable symptoms and at least half eventually require surgery. By the time men reach the age of eighty prostate problems are almost universal, although in a few cases the prostate gland atrophies with extreme age. No one knows yet why the prostate undergoes growth in midlife after a period of dormancy following adolescence. There is evidence that African-American men develop prostate enlargement an average of five years earlier than white men. There also appear to be lower rates of enlargement among non-American Asian men compared to American Asian men. Diet may be a factor, especially large amounts of fat. Some physicians believe a zinc deficiency may be involved, but there is no solid evidence for this. Zinc taken in small doses will do no harm, but it is not a medically proved treatment or preventive for prostate problems.

When the enlargement is noncancerous, as is usually the case, it is called benign prostatic hyperplasia (too many cells), or BPH. BPH starts very gradually and may exist for years with no symptoms. In fact, many men remain symptomless throughout their lives except for the enlargement. A reliable and readable book about this subject is *What Every Man Should Know About His Prostate*, revised edition by Mary-Ellen Siegel, M.S.W. (Walker and Company, 1988). Also see "Treatment Advances of Benign Prostatic Hyperplasia" by E. D. Whitehead and H. M. Nagler in *Medical Aspects of Human Sexuality* (Cahners Publishing Co., 1990), pp. 24–29.

The size of the enlarged prostate gland is less significant than the amount of obstruction it produces at the neck of the bladder. Since the prostate gland is so close to the bladder and urethra, the enlargement can produce a number of problems with urination. Men may find themselves with some or all of the following symptoms: An enlarged prostate may increase the need and urgency to urinate or to get up to void during the night. There may be a delay in starting the stream of urine, a slowness or weakness in the stream, or even a total inability to urinate. Occasionally, small amounts of blood are present in the urine and during ejaculation. (Bleeding should *always* be medically evaluated, since it could also be a symptom of cancer.) The dribbling of urine after urination is common and requires the use of paper tissues for a few minutes to catch the drops of urine. Since enlargement of the gland may lead to retention and stagnation of urine, there can also be bacterial infection. In severe and untreated cases, damage is done to the kidneys. Surgery may be necessary when a urinary shutdown occurs.

The causes of noncancerous prostatic difficulties are unknown but may be connected to genetics, to changes in endocrine levels, and/or to the aging process itself. Previous theories about changes in hormone levels seem to have been disproved at Johns Hopkins Medical School and elsewhere. A curious aspect of BPH is that it has been found in aging men and aging dogs, but in no other species. We also should mention that there is no foundation to the folklore that prostate trouble is related to "excessive" sexual activity. Indeed, evidence suggests that an active and regular sex life preserves healthy prostate functioning, while a pattern of irregular ejaculations may lead to such problems as inflammation.

Cancer of the prostate, a much more serious disorder, occurs largely in men over sixty. Its cause is still unknown. It does not appear that men with BPH have higher rates of prostate cancer than those without BPH. Most such cancers are not detected until men are in their seventies, and *cancer of the prostate is the second leading cause of cancer deaths in men*, killing 25,500 annually. The probability of developing prostate cancer in one's lifetime is about 9 percent for American men. However, if detected early, many cases can be successfully treated with surgery and/or radiation. While both methods are effective against the cancer, surgery may be more curative, especially in the younger patient. Originally radiation was thought to be more protective of potency; however, it has now been found that a significant number of men who undergo this treatment—30 to 60 percent—do experience permanent impotence.

Chemotherapy (cis-platin or vinoristine) and hormone therapy are also commonly used in the treatment of prostatic cancer. During the course of chemotherapy, problems with erections and desire may emerge, but they do disappear after the therapy has stopped. Hormone therapy involves either bilateral orchiectomy (removal of both testicles) or hormones (e.g., estrogen-type), or a combination of both. The intent of hormone therapy is to eliminate the testosterone that feeds this cancer. Side effects can include a decrease in sexual desire and difficulties in erection. However, penile injections or vacuum devices can counteract the impotence (see pages 96–99), but testosterone treatments should not be given.

Cancer of the prostate is relatively slow-growing and may go through dormant periods. A physical exam at least once a year after age forty, including a digital (finger) rectal examination (DRE) and a complete urinalysis, greatly enhances the chance of early detection. Many urologists, including the Prostate Health Program of New York, advise that the new blood test (PSA) be performed at the time of the DRE.

In 1982, a nerve-sparing operation (a modified radical retropubic prostatectomy), designed to protect the nerve centers damaged by the usual cancer surgery, was developed at Johns Hopkins by Dr. Patrick Walsh. Many urologists now offer such surgery, which preserves potency in 70 percent of those who have the operation. This nerve-sparing surgery has been incorporated into a prostate cancer operation called radical perineal prostectomy, which is rapidly gaining favor.

Advances in the medical (including hormonal) treatment of BPH also seem promising. For example, Hytrin, a brand of terazosin, relieves pressure on the urethra almost immediately and mitigates symptoms in about two-thirds of prostate patients by its effects on the muscles. It does have some untoward side effects, such as dizziness and fatigue.

And the drug Proscar not only shrinks the prostate, according to both animal studies and initial human studies, but appears to be free of major side effects. With Proscar, it takes about three months before the prostate shrinks enough to relieve symptoms. The drug specifically blocks 5-alpha reductase, the enzyme that converts testosterone to dihydrotestosterone, the hormone associated with the growth of the prostate gland. According to the results of clinical trials, more than half of the 1,600 patients studied over a twelve-month period showed at least 20 percent prostate shrinkage, and about one-third experienced significant clinical improvement. Of those treated with Proscar, 3.7 percent became impotent, whereas 1.6 percent of those on a placebo reported impotence. 3.3 percent of the Proscar subjects also reported decreased sexual desire. Impotence and lack of desire proved reversible once the patients stopped taking the drug.

Also, a new treatment for BPH that uses a laser is currently being tested. The YAG laser is an intense light beam that can be used under local anesthesia to destroy the excess prostate tissue in benign prostatic enlargement. The tissue is then voided with the urine. The advantage of the laser is that it avoids other surgical procedures and allows the extra tissue to be painlessly eliminated. This is still in its experimental stages, however, and is not yet available for the general public. There is also the balloon treatment, in which a tiny balloon is run through a catheter to the prostate gland and inflated with high pressure for several minutes, to open up the urethra. Its side effects are few, and for some, this treatment seems effective. Yet at present, a prostatectomy to treat the BPH remains the treatment of choice, with 400,000 prostatectomies being performed each year. (Twenty percent of those who undergo this surgery must undergo a second operation within ten years.) Some doctors now recommend surgery at an early point in the course of symptoms to avoid unnecessary complications and dire emergencies; this is a decision best made jointly by you and your doctor.

There are three types of prostatectomies, all of which require anesthesia:

Transurethral resection, or TUR, is the commonest, least traumatic, and safest surgical procedure because it requires no outside incision. A thin, hollow, fiber-optic tube is inserted in the penis, an electric loop is maneuvered through the tube, and the prostate gland is removed. One disadvantage of this technique is that the tissue sometimes grows back. TUR is recommended chiefly when the prostate is not too enlarged, and for men over seventy.

Suprapubic or *retropubic* surgery (named for the site of the incision, above or behind the pubic bone) is performed when the gland is very large. The tissue is removed through an incision made in the abdomen.

Perineal surgery is used by some surgeons for men with substantial prostate enlargement who are in poor physical condition. There is very little postoperative bleeding or pain with this procedure. An even more radical perineal procedure is used in the surgical treatment of cancer of the gland. These procedures can be performed with a high degree of safety even on a very elderly man. An incision is made in the perineum between the scrotum and the anus, and most or all of the prostate is removed. Whether surgery is more effective than radiotherapy for operable prostate cancer is unknown. Radiotherapy, however, results in impotence in 30 to 60 percent of men, compared to the nearly 100 percent impotence perineal surgery causes.

Potency is rarely affected by the TUR and suprapubic procedures, and some men actually experience increased potency because their prostatic problems have been eliminated. It is generally agreed that 80 percent of men return to their presurgery sexual functioning, 10 percent actually have improved sexual functioning, while 10 percent have some or even total loss of the ability to achieve an erection. (Fifteen percent of those who have had TUR experience some urinary incontinence.) The perineal approach—especially the radical procedure—has been the chief physical cause of impotence following prostatic surgery because it requires critical nerves to be cut. Perineal surgery also may affect the ability to urinate by causing strictures to form in the urethra. Dilation of the urethra is then required.

Prior to surgery, prostate problems usually do not interfere with sexual functioning unless pain is present. Some men may experience a slight decrease in the force of their ejaculation, but others may have benign prostate problems for years with no change in sexual functioning. After a prostatectomy, particularly for those operations done for BPH as we have noted, most men resume normal sexual activity. Healing time runs at least six weeks, and most men wait four to six weeks before resuming sexual activity. The only sexual change after most types of surgery is that in many cases semen is no longer ejaculated through the penis but instead is pushed backward into the bladder (retrograde ejaculation), where it is voided with the urine. This so-called dry ejaculation happens because a space has been left where the enlarged prostate had been, and fluid travels the path of least resistance to the bladder. Although men in this situation can no longer father children, the large majority have erections as before, with no diminishment of sexual pleasure. (However, if couples wish, sperm can be successfully extracted from the urine and deposited in the younger female partner's vagina for fertilization purposes.) It is important not to depend on retrograde ejaculation for birth control, however, since some semen may still pass down through the penis. In addition, normal ejaculation may very well return following some regrowth of the prostate; in such instances, fertility may be restored. (A certain amount of regrowth can occur without causing difficulties or requiring surgery.)

By far the greatest cause of impotence occurring with prostatectomies is *psychological*. Unfortunately, family doctors and urologists do not always provide adequate information about what to expect after surgery, so that a man falsely assumes sexual impairment. This assumption, with its consequent fear, is based on the tendency to associate the prostate gland with the penis, since the two are in physical proximity.

And beware of the many quack remedies that promise treatment without surgery. Various kinds of massage, foods, and other "cures," often at exorbitant prices, are offered to men seeking a quick cure for a sometimes serious condition. Avoid them and rely instead on your physician's advice.

MALE INCONTINENCE

Today there are many treatment options to help with urinary incontinence whether or not there has been surgery performed for an enlarged prostate or to treat cancer of the prostate. The implantation of a urinary prosthesis can control the flow of urine for approximately 90 percent of those men who undergo insertions of a urinary sphincter. For more information on bladder control problems, including incontinence, contact The Association for Urinary Continence Control, 785 Park Avenue, New York, New York 10021 (phone: 212-988-8888), or send a business-size SASE to HIP (Help for Incontinent People), P.O. Box 544, Union, South Carolina 29379 (phone: 803-579-7900).

ORCHIECTOMY

This surgery, which is removal of the testes, may follow cancer of the prostate. The psychological impact of this castration can be devastating. Emotional preparation before and counseling following the surgery are absolutely indispensable. The placement of artificial testes (made of plastic or tantalum) may be advisable for both cosmetic and emotional reasons. Impotence does not always follow removal of the testes; some men do continue to have normal erections. Usually ejaculations no longer occur, although there may be a little prostate fluid.

COLOSTOMY AND ILEOSTOMY

When part of the bowel must be removed for lifesaving purposes, the anus is generally closed and an artificial opening in the abdomen created. The surgery may be in the colon (colostomy) or in the ileum (an ileostomy). Needless to say, the patient has many sensitive adjustments to make after such surgery. A bag attached to the opening fills with feces and must be emptied, although many colostomy patients develop enough bowel predictability to simply wear a gauze pad. There are possible embarrassing bowel sounds as well as odors, although much of this can be adequately controlled. Those who undergo ostomies have to work their way through their own feelings, as well as their perceptions of other people's attitudes. And the most complicated issue of all can be working out the sexual relationship with one's partner. Information and counseling specific to ostomies can help greatly.

Estimates are that it may take up to a year to make a full and relatively comfortable adjustment to an ostomy. Your primary physician as well as your surgeon are central in helping you anticipate and circumvent or resolve problems. Although most are grateful that their lives have been spared by ostomies, it is normal to experience difficulties in accepting the changes in one's body. Those who had active sex lives prior to ostomies usually continue to have them afterward, but inevitably there is a complex adjustment process, and you and your partner should not hesitate to seek help. Over a million people in the United States have had ostomies, and United Ostomy Clubs have been formed, which can offer a great deal of support. For information on the local chapter nearest you (there are more than 250 nationwide), contact the United Ostomy Association, 36 Executive Park, Suite 120, Irvine, California 92714. "Sex, Courtship and the Single Ostomate" is a pamphlet available from the association.

RECTAL CANCER SURGERY

If a cancerous tumor is operable and is not in the lower two-thirds of the rectum, surgery can be done that not only permits normal bowel function but also allows normal sexual activity. However, if removal of the tumor requires removal of the rectum and anus, with a permanent colostomy, men may become totally impotent. The closeness of the male genital organs to the lower rectum leaves essential nerve fibers vulnerable to damage from such surgery. Women, on the other hand, maintain the capacity for sexual arousal and orgasm even after rectal surgery, since the essential nerves involved are farther removed from the surgical site.

IN SUMMARY

In general, for both men and women, the emotionally charged aspects of surgery and its effects on sexuality can be relatively short-lived *if* people spell out their fears and *if* their misconceptions are cleared up. Unfortunately, they often do not get the opportunity to do this. Doctors do not always take the time to explain procedures and answer questions, although counseling before surgery is extremely helpful in preventing anxiety and clarifying misunderstandings. After the operation, continued advice and emotional support from medical personnel, family, friends, and special organizations are crucial. Be sure to ask for help, and if you remain troubled, seek professional psychotherapy to work through your more complicated feelings.

Even with the best of modern techniques, rates of recovery vary with the individual after surgery of any kind. Some people find their stamina or vitality reduced for some time, even though healing has been satisfactory. These are normal variations. You have no reason to worry if this happens to you, as long as your surgeon has assured you that your postoperative recovery is progressing as it should be. Once you are feeling entirely well again, your level of sexual activity is likely to return to normal.

CHAPTER 5

❧❧❧

SEXUAL FITNESS

Sex is one of the great free and renewable pleasures of life. To get the most out of it, however, you should be in shape for it. Two powerful aphrodisiacs are a vigorous and well-cared-for body and a lively personality. Much can be done to preserve the functioning of both, although we shall be talking here specifically about your body. The overall formula for keeping in good health and preventing a multitude of problems is a simple one: no smoking, moderate use of alcohol, control of blood pressure and weight, balanced nutrition, regular exercise, and adequate rest.

FITNESS FOR OLDER PEOPLE

The enjoyment of sex is enhanced by a fairly healthy, fairly pain-free body. Apart from visits to the doctor for a specific complaint, older men and women ideally should have a physical examination every year. Women should also have a gynecological examination every six months, particularly to check for breast and vaginal cancer. Bring any problems in sexual functioning to your doctor's attention at the time of these examinations, if not at a special appointment in between. The purpose of all this is to detect and treat physical problems in their early stages and to obtain medical guidance for a program of preventive health care, including exercise, nutrition, and rest.

EXERCISE

Exercise can improve physical appearance and it can definitely increase longevity. It is crucial for a healthy heart, arteries, and respiratory system, and has a relaxing effect on the nervous system. Studies indicate that bones maintain their size and strength better during aging if one exercises regularly. In addition, exercise can improve one's sex life. The only bad news is that exercise requires discipline and a certain amount of work!

Although we are improving our habits as a nation, many Americans do not exercise at all, and older people exercise less often than younger people. This is unfortunate, since the older you are, the more help your body needs from you. So plan to exercise on a routine and daily basis.

Physical fitness is a condition of looking and feeling good and having the necessary physical reserves to enjoy a range of interests, including sex. Fitness has two components. *Organic fitness* involves basic health, a well-nourished body as free as possible from disease or infirmity, with physical limitations compensated for to the greatest degree possible. *Dynamic fitness* means not simply freedom from disease but the full ability to move vigorously and energetically. This involves efficiency of heart and lungs, muscular strength and endurance, balance, flexibility, coordination, and agility.

To reach an optimum level in both components of fitness, you need to perform two distinct kinds of exercise: one to keep the body limber and supple and strengthen the muscles (stretching, flexing, and weight-bearing exercises), the other to increase endurance and enlarge the heart capacity (aerobic exercises).

To achieve a personal level of fitness, you should exercise aerobically for at least twenty to thirty continuous minutes three to five times a week, at about 70 percent of your age-adjusted maximum heart rate. To find your maximum rate, subtract your age from 220. For example, a sixty-year-old would subtract 60 from

220, which is 160. Seventy percent of 160 would equal 112 heartbeats a minute, or about 18 beats every ten seconds. For aerobic benefits, fast walking, swimming, cycling, cross-country skiing, and skating, all of which involve continual movement, are better than basketball, dance, handball, tennis, and racquetball, which involve intermittent movement. Be wary of jogging and fast action sports like racquetball, which can cause injury to the bones and joints.

Brisk walking is perhaps the best all-around exercise for older people, especially when it is accompanied by a regimen of calisthenics. The squeezing action of the leg muscles on the veins during walking helps promote the return of blood to the heart. Start out by walking rapidly until you begin to feel tired. Rest and walk back to your starting point. Keep doing this for progressively longer distances until you reach a reasonable goal, such as a walk of two to three miles a day in forty-five minutes. (This may take a year or so if you have previously been sedentary.)

As a supplement to a regular program of exercise, take advantage of any opportunity for physical movement—walking upstairs, doing chores, mowing the lawn, gardening—in short, bending, stretching, and moving as much as possible. But don't depend on these activities alone to keep you supple. For specific stretching and strengthening exercises, see the exercise book recommended on page 149.

If you have been unusually inactive or had any

indication of possible heart disease, take a treadmill stress test (available in most hospitals) before jogging, swimming, and other more vigorous activities. Swimming is particularly useful for anyone with a joint disease like arthritis or orthopedic problems such as damaged knees or chronic backache. It is not recommended as the major physical activity to protect against osteoporosis, however, because, unlike walking, it is not weight-bearing on the long bones of the body.

The use of a stationary bicycle or a treadmill is popular with older people because they are accessible in all kinds of weather, and, if you have one of them in your home, it requires no transportation to and from exercise periods. They also allow accurate measurement of the amount of exercise you are getting. However, if you use a bicycle at home, you must have good knees and no major orthopedic problems, and you must be strongly motivated to exercise alone.

Spa fitness centers, exercise resorts, and the best aerobic centers and health clubs that are proliferating in and near major cities have begun to pay more attention to the medical as well as the aesthetic and social aspects of exercise. The most medically oriented of such programs are those found at the Duke University Diet and Fitness Center in Durham, North Carolina, and the Pritikin Longevity Centers, one located near Los Angeles and the other in Miami Beach. These programs offer superb health education, individualized diet and exercise programs, and behavioral training to change old habits and take on new ones. Canyon Ranch, located in both Tucson, Arizona, and Lexington, Massachusetts, also has developed a well-run fitness program. Unfortunately, all these centers tend to be very expensive.

Most spas and fitness centers today are coed, and men must be warned that they will usually not be able to achieve the same level of flexibility as most women. This is not a sign that they are not trying hard enough. It simply means that male and female bodies are different, and women are generally more flexible than men. On the other hand, men often have a natural advantage over women in exercises that emphasize strength. Ideally, both men and women should approach exercise noncompetitively. In fact, precisely because there are wide variations in physical performance and capacity, your own individual physical condition should determine the exercise appropriate for you and its level and pace. If you become temporarily ill or inactive, you will usually need to return to an earlier level of activity and slowly work your way back up. In all cases, avoid strenuous bursts of sudden activity when you are out of shape. We also recommend that you discuss your exercise program with your doctor and ask him or her to advise you.

Some people don't exercise out of the fear that it will provoke a heart attack. What they do not realize is that exercise *opposes* the effect of stroke or heart attack. Blood clots form when the blood is sluggish rather than when it is circulating vigorously. A now-classic study of

17,000 middle-aged and older Harvard alumni over several years by Dr. Ralph Paffenbarger and colleagues, published in the *Journal of the American Medical Association,* July 27, 1984, found a greater risk of coronary heart disease among those who led sedentary life-styles. As described in Chapter 3, people who have had heart attacks are usually placed on an exercise program by their physicians shortly after their initial recovery in order to reduce the possibility of another attack. Exercise is also valuable for preventing and treating hypertension, diabetes, and osteoporosis.

A growing number of exercise books are being written specifically for older people, including those who are wheelchair-bound or bedridden. A good book for those in their middle and later years is *Biomarkers: The Ten Keys to Prolonging Vitality* by William Evans and Irwin Rosenberg, with Jacqueline Thompson (Fireside/Simon and Schuster, 1991).

Exercising Your Trouble Spots.

There are specific exercises that can greatly improve your appearance if they are undertaken on a regular basis.

A *protruding abdomen* can be controlled by dieting and by regularly performing exercises which strengthen both the upper and lower abdominal muscles.

The upper abdomen is strengthened by exercises called *crunches*. To start, lie on your back on a thick rug or exercise mat on the floor. Bend your knees so that your feet rest flat on the floor. Put your hands behind your head. Use your upper abdominal muscles to raise your shoulders off the floor in a forward curling motion. Then slowly lower your shoulders back to the floor again. Repeat this movement ten to twelve times in one set. Start with one set per day, building up gradually to three sets per day. Take a rest of about one to two minutes between sets.

The lower abdomen is exercised by *knee raises*. To start, lie flat on your back on the floor on a rug or exercise mat. Place your hands, palms down, under your buttocks. Bend your knees so that your feet are flat on the floor. Use your lower abdominal muscles to slowly raise your feet off the floor and bring your knees up to your chest. Then slowly bring your feet back to the floor to the starting position. Repeat movement as directed for *crunches,* described above.

Improving *back muscles* will help your stomach muscles, as well as prevent or alleviate back pain. As much as 80 percent of backaches are due to muscle fatigue rather than slipped discs or arthritis. Lie on your back, squeeze your buttocks together, and tighten stomach muscles while flattening your back against the floor. Hold for a count of five, then relax. Repeat ten times. Swimming is also excellent for those with back problems.

In later years many women develop *weakened pelvic muscles,* which makes them feel their vagina is losing its gripping ability. The Kegel exercises for women consist of contractions of the muscles of the pelvic floor, as though one were holding oneself back from urinating and defecating at the same time. It should be possible to feel the muscles tightening. Perform these exercises several times daily while in either a sitting or standing position. Hold the contraction for only a few seconds each time. The process must be repeated daily for at least one hundred contractions for the Kegel exercises to be truly effective.

Many women find the Kegel exercises difficult because they find it hard to focus on exercising the correct muscles. One helpful device women can use is the Femina Cone. When inserted into the vagina, the smooth plastic weighted cone will tend to slip out unless the proper muscles are contracted. This helps women learn which muscles to contract for Kegel exercises. For more information on Femina Cones, write Dacomed, Inc., 1701 East 79th St., Minneapolis, MN 55425.

When there is improved muscle tone as a result of using the Kegel exercises, the vaginal walls also then exert greater pressure on the penis. This is of particular value in those older couples where the man's penis has become somewhat smaller and the woman's vagina larger. Some women are able to use the Kegel movement in a rhythmic fashion during sexual intercourse, thus increasing both partners' satisfaction. The exercises also help to support the pelvic structure—the

uterus, bladder, and rectum. Some physicians even prescribe Kegel exercises for men, to treat or prevent prostatitis.

POSTURE

The last word on posture is to stand tall (yes, your
mother was right), although not in the ramrod posture
popular in military training. Stand firmly on your two
feet and then extend your head up as far as comfortably
possible; the rest of the body, including the spine, will
then tend to fall correctly in a relaxed alignment. It may
require vigilance to remember this stance, especially if
you are attempting to change years of bad posture habits. But the "stand tall" mind-set can be nurtured
through yoga, such body therapies as the Alexander
Method, and personal training with health professionals
skilled in body mechanics and alignment.

NUTRITION

If you are over sixty, beware of poor nutrition and even
malnutrition. You may protest, "That's absurd! I've always eaten a normal diet." Well, poor nutrition can
creep up on you in later life. Medical and lay people

alike share the illusion that the United States is the world's best-fed nation, but "overfed" is more accurate. The United States has the highest percentage of overweight people in the world, and poor nutrition is widespread, even among those who eat large amounts of food.

This state of affairs is especially true when it comes to older people. There are many reasons for this, the most obvious being the rising cost of good-quality food and the lowered incomes of many people, especially women, as they grow older. But there are other, less obvious reasons. Social isolation and depression can cause people to lose their appetite and stop taking an interest in cooking; physical limitations may make shopping and preparing food difficult; loss of teeth or poor teeth interfere with eating solid foods; illnesses, alcoholism, and chronic diseases of many kinds can affect food consumption; and finally, poor eating habits may develop (snacking, the tea-and-toast syndrome, and use of junk and convenience foods). Those who live alone are especially prone to neglect a proper diet—"It's too much bother to fix a meal for just one person."

What are the dangers of poor nutrition? First, you become more vulnerable to disease. You get fatigued more easily and lose your sense of well-being. You are also more likely to have emotional problems, among them depression, apathy, and anxiety. Age-related processes can be accelerated, and sexual interest and performance are often lowered. In other words, there are a host of reasons to eat well, aside from enjoying the taste of food itself.

How can you embark on a healthy, nutritious diet? A healthy diet includes three kinds of food groups—carbohydrates (cereals, breads, vegetables, fruits), proteins (meat, dairy products, eggs, fish, poultry, beans, nuts, and some grains), and fats (meat, dairy products, oils, nuts, and grains).

Carbohydrates, the complex starches and natural sugars in fruits, vegetables, and grains, are emerging as the healthiest foods overall, supplemented by poultry, fish, and low-fat dairy products. You should strictly limit your intake of red meat, any kind of animal or dairy fat, and egg yolks. Refined carbohydrates are often the most tempting foods, and both sweet tooths, who love sugar, and people who find starchy foods irresistible may overload their diets with them. Refined starches, sugar, and other sweeteners fill the stomach, raise the blood sugar, lower the appetite, and lead to a false sense of well-being. Do not be deceived. *You must have some proteins every day for vitality and body-tissue repair.* If cost is a problem, learn more about preparing foods "from scratch" using low-cost proteins (dried skim milk, dried beans, cheaper cuts of meat, etc.). The home economics departments of high schools or colleges near you can offer advice, as will the U.S. Department of Agriculture. Write to the Superintendent of Documents, Government Printing Office, Washington, DC 20402 for nutrition information. In general, it is wise to cut down on desserts, pastries, fatty meats, gravies, beer, sweet wines, hard liquors, and soft drinks. Use vegetable oils and margarines that are low in saturated fats, and try to eliminate butter, lard, cream, and margarines high in saturated fats.

If you happen to be overweight and need to diet, good general references are *Jane Brody's Nutrition Book* (Norton, 1982), *Jane Brody's Good Food Book* (Bantam, 1987), *Dr. Dean Ornish's Program for Reversing Heart Disease* (Ballantine Books, 1990), and Robert Pritikin's *The New Pritikin Program: The Easy and Delicious Way to Shed Fat, Lower Your Cholesterol and Stay Fit* (Simon and Schuster, 1990). Avoid crash and fad diets since they can harm your health and your appearance. Develop food habits you can live with comfortably, in good health, while still losing weight. Supplementing a sensible weight loss diet with regular aerobic exercise is the surest way to lose weight and keep that weight off. Diet clubs such as TOPS, Weight Watchers, and Overeaters Anonymous, or self-organized dieting clubs can make it easier for people with persistent weight problems to lose pounds.

Diets aimed at the prevention of disease are important far before age sixty. We know a good deal, for example, about diet and the prevention and control of heart disease. The earliest of the heart disease prevention diets is the Prudent Man's Diet, devised by Dr. Norman Jolliffe in 1957. This was a balanced, low-calorie diet that called for a total of 2,400 calories a day (compared to the American male's average of 3,200), with no more than 30 percent fat, a cholesterol limit of 300 mg a day (roughly the amount in one egg), moderate protein, increased complex carbohydrates such as vegetables and fruits, and a reduction of salt.

Epidemiological cross-national data now exist that relate health and longevity with even lower-fat diets (e.g., in China, only 10 percent of calories in the daily diet is in the form of fat). The Pritikin and Ornish diets mentioned earlier call for individuals to eat only 10 percent of daily calories in fat, while the American Heart Association recommends a maximum of 30 percent. We personally would suggest drawing the line at 20 percent, as this is a difficult enough target. The new FDA food labeling system will help you in calculating this target. You can also obtain low-fat recipes and cooking advice from your local heart association or from the American Heart Association, 205 East 42nd Street, New York, New York 10017. *The Long Life Cookbook* by Anne Casale (Ballantine Books, 1988) is also a good source of recipes and information.

To help you become more aware about the dangers and benefits of cholesterol, look at the following information:

• The average blood cholesterol for all Americans today is 210 mg. For older people, a cholesterol level of 240–260 mg (per deciliter of blood) indicates moderate risk of heart attack, while levels above 260 mg are at high risk.

• A specific subfraction of high density lipoprotein (HDL) cholesterol, called HDL_2, may actually protect against heart attack. Recent studies indicate that an extended program of regular aerobic exercise raises HDL_2.

• Fatty fish, such as salmon and mackerel, and monounsaturated fats, such as olive oil, may have cholesterol-lowering effects.

• Nearly all clinical trials of the effects of cholesterol lowering have focused on middle-aged men. We know less about women and even less about the elderly. Some feel that those who are very old and frail should not restrict their cholesterol intake because of the risk of not eating enough to meet their caloric and nutritional needs.

Other specific nutritional tips for those of you who are older:

• Go easy on salt, since you are more susceptible to high blood pressure.

• Bulk in your diet is very important for digestion. This is true for all older people but especially for those who are dieting to lose weight. Doctors used to prescribe low-residue (limited-bulk) diets for older people with bowel problems, but now just the opposite is generally true. Bulk can be obtained by eating fruits and vegetables (complex carbohydrates) like raw celery, apples, and carrots, as well as whole-grain bread and cereals. Bran cereal is also a good choice. If you want lots of bulk at low cost, buy coarse bran (local health-food stores usually carry it) for a few cents a pound. If you don't live near a health-food store, get a mail-order health-food catalog. Coarse bran tastes like a cross between babies' pabulum and sawdust (in other words—not so good!), but if you take several teaspoonfuls in between swallows of fruit juice at each meal or a larger amount on your breakfast cereal daily, you will be taking an important step in promoting good bowel action and preventing diverticulosis, certain kinds of constipation, and other bowel problems. Bran is *far* better for you than laxatives. And the complex carbohydrates may be even better.

• Try to avoid getting into the habit of taking laxatives, which can in fact induce habitual constipation. As we have noted, a good diet with plenty of bulk, plenty of exercise, and plenty of fluids (8 glasses a day) are the best ways to prevent constipation. If you do need an occasional laxative, many doctors feel that milk of magnesia is preferable to mineral oil, which tends to reduce the absorption of fat-soluble vitamins.

• "Indigestion" from eating fried foods may mean gallstones, so consult your doctor. Some liver specialists believe that a low-fat diet can help prevent the formation of gallstones.

• Gout, arthritis, diabetes, and a number of other diseases that can directly affect your sex life as well as your general health may require a special diet prescribed by your doctor.

• Some people—more often women than men— have a bumpy kind of fat known as cellulite on their thighs and hips; it resembles the texture of the skin of an orange. It can hang from upper arms or droop around the stomach, and dieting alone will not remove it. In fact, there are no reliable techniques for getting rid of this bothersome fat, but exercise and diet can help over time.

• Many older people probably would benefit from taking a standard vitamin-and-mineral supplement daily. For the average healthy individual, a multivitamin should contain no more than 100 to 150 percent of the U.S. Recommended Daily Allowance (RDA) for any one nutrient.

• Anemia (reduced hemoglobin and/or red blood cells) may occur when your diet is inadequate in iron and protein. Foods containing iron are lean meats, dark green leafy vegetables, and whole grain and enriched breads and cereals. Altering your diet to provide for the adequate amounts of iron and protein is more economical and just as effective as the highly advertised vitamin-and-mineral preparations. (Remember: your anemia should be evaluated by your doctor.)

• Osteoporosis, a common disorder, is due to a gradual loss of calcium from the bones, and its development is accelerated in women by the onset of menopause. Wrist and hip fractures and deformities such as a hump on the back may develop. High protein and salt intake, cigarette smoking, heavy caffeine and alcohol intake, lack of exercise, and a family history of osteoporosis all work toward increasing the risk of osteoporosis. The disorder may be slowed in some by adequate nutrition and exercise, although specific recommendations for doing so are still under debate. For example, opinions differ on the significance of calcium intake, with some believing that an excess of protein in the diet may be even more significant than insufficient calcium in the development of osteoporosis. Currently estrogen replacement therapy is considered the most effective treatment, but because of its possible risks, such therapy should be individualized by you and your doctor (see Chapter 2).

Efforts to prevent osteoporosis should begin in childhood and youth, with an emphasis on exercise, calcium intake, and avoidance of smoking. But you can still help to slow or delay osteoporosis starting in your middle years by increasing your calcium to an adequate intake of 1,000 milligrams before menopause and 1,500 milligrams after it. (The average intake of adult women is 450–500 milligrams a day—far too low.) About five eight-ounce glasses of skim milk (to avoid fat intake) would supply 1,500 milligrams of calcium. If you don't like milk or it does not agree with you, you should take calcium supplements containing carbonate. However, Tums, a good source of calcium carbonate, causes constipation for some. An alternative is orange juice fortified with calcium citrate. Other good sources of calcium include such foods as yogurt, hard cheese (especially Parmesan and Swiss—but do use these sparingly), canned salmon and sardines (you should eat the bones too), kidney and pinto beans, bean curd, oysters, and collard, turnip, and mustard greens.

If you are postmenopausal, be careful not to take more than the recommended amount of 1,500 milligrams; calcium in larger doses can have harmful effects. Those of you taking additional estrogen can scale back to a normal pre-menopausal dosage of 1,000 milligrams daily. Moreover, those with a tendency to develop kidney stones, ulcers, or other digestive disorders may react adversely to high calcium intake.

• Large doses of vitamin E have been recommended for a variety of disorders, including sterility and vascular diseases, and for retarding the aging process, curing impotence, and healing wounds and burns. There is as yet no definitive scientific evidence for these claims, but anecdotal evidence for certain conditions is widespread. The recommended daily allowance for women is 20 to 25 international units (IU) and for men 30 IU, although up to 400 IU per day is not thought to be harmful.

• In general, be prudent about taking over-the-counter medications widely advertised on television and radio; they are sometimes valueless, often costly, and on occasion—especially if you take them in large quantities or combine them—hazardous. An office visit to your doctor may prove less expensive as well as better for your health than self-diagnosis and self-administered remedies for a physical complaint.

• It is a common belief that people need fewer calories as they grow older. One source claims that your body will require 10 percent fewer calories between ages thirty-five and fifty-five than when you were under thirty-five, 16 percent fewer between ages fifty-five and seventy-five, and 1 percent fewer calories per year for every year over seventy-five. We are not totally convinced of this. We suspect that this theory is based on the fact that many older people become less active and fail to work or exercise their bodies, and that caloric needs are a function of activity and not of age. (Some inactivity is of course related to physical ailments, but much more is simply lack of motivation and inertia.) The older you get, the more temptation you will feel to take it easy. Remember the maxim "Most people don't wear out, they rust out." Lack of movement leads to poor appetite, which in turn leads to fatigue and a vicious cycle.

• Experts tend to believe that it is harder to lose weight as we grow older, and some say this is especially true for women. Therefore it is critical to practice a lifelong pattern of prudent eating and regular exercise.

• If you make your evening meal relatively light, you will find that you feel and sleep better. (Breakfast is the best time to eat heartily.) Cutting down on food and alcohol intake before bed is also conducive to better sex. If you do find yourself having a heavy evening meal, it would be best to postpone lovemaking for a few hours to avoid unnecessary strain on the heart and other organs.

REST

A rested body enhances sexual desire, improves sexual performance, and contributes to general health and well-being. Contrary to general opinion, as you grow older you will need as much sleep as when you were younger, or maybe even more. You may, however, notice changes in your sleep patterns. Studies show that older people seem to experience less deep or delta sleep (the period of dreamless oblivion), becoming lighter sleepers, with more frequent awakenings. In addition, depression, anxiety, grief, loneliness, and lack of exercise can affect both sleep patterns and depth of sleep. Early morning awakening is more common among the inactive, the depressed, those who go to bed early, and those who frequently take long naps during the day.

Get seven or more hours of sleep a night, according to your own personal needs. The amount of sleep needed varies from person to person, and you will find you need more sleep if you have physical health problems. If this applies to you, take one or more brief naps or rest breaks during the day, but limit total nap time to 60 to 90 minutes to avoid interfering with nighttime rest.

If insomnia strikes, don't panic. To be your most receptive for sleep, avoid caffeine drinks such as coffee, tea, and colas before bedtime—or better yet, after mid-day—since they can keep you awake. Drinking decaffeinated coffee is preferable, although some report that even the minimal amount of caffeine it contains can keep them awake. To get psychologically ready for sleep, you may want to establish these simple rituals: warm baths, firm and comfortable bed and pillows, back massage by a partner, reading a book, watching TV, or listening to music. Often warm milk, a glass of wine, or a soothing talk with your partner or an understanding friend can comfort and relax you. Exercise too can have a positive effect on sleep if completed early enough in the day, particularly if it has been performed on a regular basis for at least two months. But avoid exercising for two hours before bedtime, so that insomnia does not develop from the recent stimulation of your body.

Bedtime is a time when your defenses against anxiety, anger, and other emotions are lowered. If these emotions routinely create troubled sleep or insomnia, you may find that psychotherapy or some other form of counseling may help. Go out of your way to avoid non-prescription sleep remedies; they are expensive and, on the whole, useless. Eventually your body will become tired enough to sleep all by itself! For occasional insomnia, one or two aspirin before bed are helpful for some people. We don't recommend sleeping pills (hypnotics) unless you are in pain or great physical or emotional discomfort; they can be habit-forming and may cause adverse side effects, including, paradoxically, the perpetuation of insomnia. If you do use sleeping pills, ensure that your use of them is evaluated by your physician on an ongoing basis—these prescriptions should not be automatically renewed. Engaging in active, pleasurable sexual activity, including sexual self-stimulation, is an excellent way of inducing sleep. The effect is strongest when you have an orgasm, but even without it you will find that such activity is usually mildly relaxing.

When it comes to serious sleep disturbances and disorders, contact your physician. You may be able to find specialists in sleep disorders in your area by contacting the National Sleep Foundation, 122 S. Robertson Blvd., Suite 201, Los Angeles, California 90048.

HEARING PROBLEMS

One out of every four older people has a hearing impairment. For various reasons—among them embarrassment, pride, and a psychological determination to deny the fact—a surprising number of people refuse to use hearing aids even when these aids will help. Not all hearing impairments can be improved by wearing a hearing aid, but only an audiologist (a specialist trained in a program accredited by the American Speech and Hearing Association) or an otologist or otolaryngologist (doctors specifically trained to treat ear disorders) can determine this; if you suspect you have some hearing loss, you should consult with one of these specialists. Remember, too, that hearing impairments tend to develop gradually, so you may be unaware this is happening to you. If you find yourself frequently missing parts of ordinary conversation around you or have trouble making out the dialogue when you go to the movies, it is a good idea to have your hearing checked.

Impaired hearing isolates you from society far more than you realize. Present-day hearing aids are much less conspicuous, disfiguring, and cumbersome than they used to be, and observers are very likely to be matter-of-fact about them. If yours is the type of loss that can be compensated for by the use of a hearing aid, do not let personal inhibitions stop you from using one! You will realize how much you have been missing only after your hearing improves.

It will take time for you to accustom yourself to a hearing aid, so be prepared for an adjustment period; stick with it despite your initial discomfort, and thereafter always use your aid whenever you are with another person.

Be very careful to deal only with a responsible supplier. This is a field full of high-pressure door-to-door salesmen offering "low" prices, "easy" installment payments, and defective or shoddy equipment. It is important that you be properly tested and fitted with an aid of good quality, one that is appropriate to your needs.

People who have the kind of hearing loss that cannot be helped by a hearing aid *must* be frank with friends and intimates. It is unlikely that they will find your disclosure embarrassing; the awkwardness is more likely to be on your side. Sit close to your companion so you can hear what is being said and speak up when you do not. It is only when you attempt to conceal a hearing impairment that problems are likely to arise.

SKIN CARE FOR MEN AND WOMEN

Ideally, prevention of skin problems should begin in the early years for both men and women, but good skin care can help at *any* time in life. Skin can be damaged by too much sun or wind and by malnutrition, excess alcohol, disease, depression, drugs, and anxiety. Overexposure to the sun causes more premature aging—particularly in Caucasians—than any other factor. Sunbathing and working or playing out-of-doors unprotected for long periods of time are the major culprits. They can result in permanent skin damage affecting both the outer and inner layers of skin, causing loss of water and elasticity, deep wrinkles, and grooves. Prolonged exposure to very cold weather, overheated rooms with minimal humidity, and air conditioning in warm climates can deplete the moisture in the skin, making it look lined. Electric blankets left on all night can dry the body skin. Various kinds of air pollution can be damaging as well. Poor nutrition, whether vitamin deficiencies or unbalanced diets, can cause dry, scaly, and inelastic skin. Sagging skin sometimes follows too rapid weight loss. Anxiety, depression, and tension also speed up the appearance of aging. Cigarette smoking can cause wrinkles to appear sooner than they normally would, since nicotine narrows the small capillaries and cuts down the supply of blood bringing nourishment and oxygen to the skin. The result, often called "smoker's face," includes deep vertical wrinkles from the corners of lips or eyes; facial gauntness; and a grayish pallor.

Even with the best of preventive care, the human face begins to acquire noticeable lines and wrinkles around the age of forty. At this time there is a gradual and permanent loss of elasticity in both the skin and the underlying tissue. Wrinkles per se should not become an obsessive concern; looking your age does not mean looking unattractive. But all of us—even those not enmeshed in the cult of youth—want to look our best. Just don't waste your money on "wrinkle removers" and other gimmicks "guaranteed" to make you look younger; anything that keeps the skin moist will help to slow down the appearance of aging.

Here is a simple regimen that you can follow to take care of your skin. The first step involves thoroughly cleansing the face and neck. Many older people can tolerate a mild, super fatted soap like Dove if it is used quickly and rinsed off completely. Neutrogena, which is much more expensive than many common soaps, is also a possibility, or a rinsable cleanser, which combines cream and a small amount of soap in lotion form. (Creams and oils used alone are difficult to remove, so the skin is never completely cleansed.) After cleansing and a thorough rinsing with warm water, pat your face dry and immediately protect it with a light moisturizer by day or a heavier oily cream for night while the skin still holds the moisture absorbed from the rinse. Most inexpensive creams like Pond's work as well as the expensive ones. (Cosmetics and creams can be purchased at a reduced price through the pharmacy service provided for members of the American Association of Retired Persons. For information write NRTA-AARP Pharmacy, 1909 K Street, N.W., Washington, DC 20006.) About once a week, women might rub something rough on their faces such as cleansing grains or inexpensive cornmeal on a wet washcloth. This helps remove the outer layer of dry flaky cells. (Men need not do this, since shaving accomplishes the same purpose.)

Protect the skin on your body against drying by using a body lotion immediately after a bath or shower when the skin has absorbed moisture.

Electric facial saunas dry out the skin. The face should really not be massaged, but if you must do it, never stretch or pull the skin in any downward direction. Various chemical processes and dermabrasion (removal of the tissues of the outer skin layer with a rotating wire brush) can be dangerous unless done by skilled operators. They are also expensive. Plastic surgery (face-lifts) for both men and women can correct severe skin sagging, but they, too, are expensive, and good results last only three to five years. The best skin care advice we have for you is sensible cleansing, good diet, rest and lack of tension, and avoidance of cigarette smoking and too much sun, wind, and alcohol.

CHAPTER 6

❧ ❦

COMMON EMOTIONAL PROBLEMS WITH SEX

Upsetting events in our life—the death of a loved one, retirement, relationship conflicts, or simply too much stress and worry—can cause sexual problems. And growing older itself can be frightening, expecially if you don't know what to expect or how to handle it. Your early life experiences and society's attitudes also have an impact on how you handle your sexuality. Let's delve a little deeper into these areas.

PERSONAL ANXIETIES

A major emotional problem older men face is the *fear* of sexual impotence. While some men have to deal with actual impotence, it is a condition that is usually temporary. In fact, *impotence occurs occasionally in nearly all men of all ages* for a variety of reasons—among them fatigue, tension, illnesses, and excessive drinking. In most cases the potency returns by itself without specific treatment when the causative physical or emotional condition is reversed. In later life, however, certain men do begin to have chronic difficulty in obtaining and maintaining an erection or find that their capacity for sexual intercourse is greatly diminished or disappears completely. We discussed the possible organic causes of impotence in Chapter 3, but it is unwise to overlook the fact that many problems can also have psychological foundations. The sex organs are a barometer of a man's feelings and quickly reflect his state of mind and current life situation. In fact, the nerve connections that control the penis are extremely sensitive to emotions. Anxiety, fear, and anger are the primary feelings that can cause a man to lose an erection rapidly—or fail to achieve one in the first place. So a disturbance in sexual functioning is often one of the first indications of unusual stress or emotional problems.

Men who do not know about the *normal* physiological changes in their sexual behavior that come with aging may believe falsely that they are becoming impotent. The expectation of high performance, which is taught to males from childhood on through constant emphasis on competition and winning, leads many men to overemphasize the physical-performance aspect of their sexuality. They become focused on erections and ejaculations rather than on expressing their feelings. This makes impotence or even its threat greatly upsetting. Thus the very *fear* of impotence can *cause* impotence. The harder a man tries to have an erection, the less likely he is to succeed. Impotence does not respond to will power and force. And if it is truly transitory, it is much more likely to improve with relaxation and freedom from pressure.

Unresponsive sexual partners can threaten men and lead to impotence. A woman's disinterest or perfunctory acquiescence is very likely to affect her partner. Women may also become impatient or demanding and make a transitory potency problem more severe. Some even find the impotence threatening to their own self-esteem and react with hostility or hurt: they see it as a sign of disinterest in them or a failure on their part to be sexually attractive.

Emotional and physical fatigue, boredom with routine lovemaking, overwork, and worries about family or finances can all affect potency. Impotence is often one of the first symptoms of depression. Disappointment, sadness, and grief over personal losses can be factors. So can resentfulness and irritation.

Sometimes impotence results from an unrecognized fear of death or injury. Fred, a businessman and retired army officer, had been a vigorous and sexually active man until he suffered a coronary attack at age seventy-two. After the attack he was unable to have an erection. It took many sessions with a psychiatrist to help him recognize that his *fear* of sexual activity triggering another coronary was the reason he did not allow himself to have an erection. His doctors suggested a provisional program of exercise, including sex, that would not jeopardize his heart. As Fred's anxiety lessened through psychotherapeutic counseling, and his sense of well-being increased as a result of his physical fitness program, his sexual ability returned.

A sudden attack of impotence is likely to be the result of some unusual stress and, once the stress is relieved, will usually abate. Even if you've experienced a lack of potency for quite some time, all you may need to overcome your condition might be information and reassurance from a doctor or professional counselor. If you find the impotence still persists, however, you may require a comprehensive medical evaluation and more extended psychotherapy and/or sexual counseling. Through this all, it is important to recognize that your partner's support plays a critical role in your overcoming your impotence.

Women are somewhat less subject to the fear of sexual dysfunctioning in later life than men, mainly because they do not have to worry about erection. Except for possible menopausal changes, the normal physical changes that accompany aging interfere very little with a woman's sexual ability. Unlike most men, women can perform the sex act even when they are emotionally upset or uninterested. While they may not enjoy love-making or have an orgasm in these situations, they are physically capable of having intercourse. (One worry women may have is about orgasmic capacity, much as men are concerned about erection and ejaculatory capacity.) Indeed, in later life some women become more relaxed about sex and come to enjoy it more, once menopause has freed them from their fear of unwanted pregnancies. Their lives may also become less pressured, their responsibilities diminishing after their children leave home; in this way the "empty nest" frequently becomes a welcome event rather than a problem.

But women can and do have other problems. Many older men and women grew up believing that "nice" women were not interested in sex and indeed found it distasteful. Women were traditionally admonished or conditioned to be passive, resigned, and accepting; it was only "loose" women who gave themselves to the pleasures of sex or sought it. A nineteenth-century marriage manual advised: "As a general rule, a modest woman seldom desires any sexual gratification for herself. She submits to her husband, but only to please him; and, but for the desire of maternity, would far rather be relieved from his attentions." Women may even remember being taught that sex was simply a duty. Men were the pursuers, women were reluctant and pursued. Such ingrained attitudes can easily interfere with developing close relationships in which both partners openly share in the enjoyment of sex. If this has been your experience, speak frankly about these issues with your partner, to clear up these antiquated assumptions. If you find it necessary, seek professional help.

The most profound emotional and sexual difficulties older women face revolve around the possibility of finding themselves alone—widowed, divorced, separated, or single—as they grow older. Their lives are affected by one major fact: there are not enough men to go around. In the United States in 1990 there were 12.5 million men aged sixty-five or over, and 18.6 million women. This disparity increases year by year as time passes, for two reasons. First, women outlive men by an average of seven years. (In 1989 life expectancy from birth was 78.6 years for females and 71.8 years for males, according to the Census Bureau.) Second, women marry men an average of three years older than themselves. And in 1990, of the 18.6 million women over sixty-five, 8.5 million were widowed and 1.8 million were divorced or single. This all adds up to the fact that 60 percent of older women are on their own, an interesting fact when one considers that they, more than any younger group, were raised from childhood to consider themselves dependent on men.

THE "OLD-PERSON" TRAP

Even when their physical and mental health is excellent, men and women in their fifties, sixties, and seventies sometimes exhibit an old-man or old-woman act, as though they were tottering invalids on their last legs. They have a rigid, stereotyped, desexualized image of what an older person *should* be, and play the role with stubborn determination. Playing the "old-person act" allows them to avoid responsibility toward themselves and others and to evoke sympathy. It can be a symbol of a perverse reluctance to "grow up" into a mature old age, or it can be simply a sign of demoralization and giving up.

Many simply decide their sexual ability is gone and arbitrarily declare themselves to be sexually incapacitated. They typically refuse to discuss the issue with their partner or to even consider possible remedies. What lies behind these actions is an attempt to avoid any type of anxiety about sex or a sexual relationship.

Such was the case with Paul, age seventy-two, a classic example of someone playing the old-person act. He shuffled along with his head bent and body slouched—in spite of the fact that he was in perfect health. He also had both a supportive wife and family, and was financially secure. So why *was* he acting this way? Paul denied that he was doing anything, but his wife claimed it was because he was angry and depressed at growing old. Paul didn't try to help himself overcome this attitude. The outcome? His wife ended up losing respect for him, and eventually her interest in him sexually waned.

Many believe they have become ugly and undesirable and begin to hate the way they look as a result of the aging process. They make frantic attempts to appear young, and end up becoming depressed at the futility of altering their appearance significantly. This was how Marlena felt. Whenever she looked in the mirror she could see the thickening in her thighs. She tried to control her eating, but even after she lost ten pounds, her legs failed to regain their former shape. She tried many supposed cures and embarked on a low-impact aerobics course. Nothing helped. It got to the point that Marlena made her partner Jim turn off the lights whenever they made love. She simply could not believe that he would be interested in her if he saw how she "truly" looked.

Another variation of this kind of self-hatred is found in those who look into the mirror and insist that what they see "is not the real me." They may decide that their only true self is interior, and refuse to accept or identify with their physical characteristics. It may take some time, but they must eventually accept the realities of change.

Sometimes older people angrily respond to their own sexual and social deprivation with hostility toward those who are younger. Everyone has heard bitter threats such as "You'll see what it's like when *you're* old" or "Wait until you reach *my* age—you won't be so smart." They might even offer self-righteous criticism of the sexuality of their own contemporaries as well as of the young.

It's vital that you recognize that you *can* make a self-fulfilling prophecy of sexual failure. Don't let yourself be overwhelmed and demoralized by the unattractive picture society draws of late life, so that you literally give up without trying, or guarantee your own failure when you do try. *To anticipate failure is to cause it to happen.* If you think you are unattractive, you tend to become so. If you believe you are sexually ineligible, you are likely to hide from those opportunities that might lead to social and sexual encounters.

So how can you avoid the old-person trap? One of the best cures is to find lively and attractive older persons with whom you can associate and identify. They provide invaluable role models when you are just beginning to search out satisfying ways to live your own life. Talk to them, ask their advice, and try on new behaviors. And when you are ready, take on the responsibility of being a role model to others.

SEXUAL GUILT AND SHAME

Sexual guilt and shame play a role in many people's reaction to sex. These feelings derive from childhood and family experiences, and from the sexual searchings of childhood, which can so often be confusing and disturbing. People past sixty, often brought up in a period

179

of Victorian-like prudery, are likely to have been treated to more than their share of misinformation, made to feel guilty about any sexual stirrings they sensed, and given few chances to get satisfying answers to their questions—if they dared ask them in the first place. The culture at that time insisted that childhood was innocent of sexuality, and any normal expression of it—looking, feeling, talking, touching—was often punished.

Masturbation itself was strictly forbidden. The Victorians even invented a grotesque array of mechanical devices to make certain that children, particularly boys, would not be able to stimulate themselves. Indeed, children were warned that masturbation could cause feeblemindedness or madness; it could "use up the life juices," weaken the body and shorten the life span, and make one nervous, distracted, and highstrung. Dark circles under the eyes were alleged indications of secret masturbation, and a grisly folklore sprang up in which hands withered and fell off if they were used in sexual stimulation.

An important misassumption that many older men still have from their youth is that "too much" sexual activity reduces potency and lowers semen "reserves." The belief that semen must be conserved is sheer nonsense because it is constantly produced—yet as late as 1945 the *Boy Scout Manual* warned youths not to "waste vital fluids."

Because for older men and women the greater part of their procreative years occurred before birth control techniques were as sophisticated, reliable, and freely available as they are today, spontaneous sexual enjoyment was often hampered by the fear of pregnancy and justified fears of venereal disease, for which effective drugs had not yet been devised. Many traditional religious teachings also imposed psychological inhibitions on sexuality.

These teachings still exert an influence on older people today. A woman in her seventies wrote:

> I feel guilty about having sexual relations with a man I'm not married to. Carl and I are both widowed, in our early seventies, and have known each other for thirty years. Every month we spend a few days at each other's home.
>
> Carl says we shouldn't feel guilty at our age and that he would like to marry me. Although I enjoy our relationship, I don't want to remarry. I've been widowed twice, most recently four years ago. Do you see any harm in my relationship with Carl?

Often it is hard for older people to give themselves freely to sexual expression. It is not easy to overcome ingrained guilt and shame even when your better judgment tells you that sexuality need no longer be considered evil or dangerous (keeping in mind, of course, that if you are not in a strictly monogamous relationship you must practice "safer sex" as a precaution against the scourge of AIDS). Thinking through your own childhood and early adult experiences may help you understand your present feelings better. Such feelings may initially be difficult to resolve, but remember once again that sexual problems, whether caused by personal or by social factors, are rarely insurmountable if approached with determination and accurate information.

PROBLEMS BETWEEN PARTNERS

If you are experiencing problems in your relationship with your sexual partner, these can very quickly affect your sexual functioning. An angry, bored, or otherwise unresponsive partner can lead to potency problems for men and sexual disinterest or lack of response for women.

Low sexual interest rather than impotence per se may be a central problem for many men. Dr. Joseph LoPiccolo believes that a chronic low sex drive is much more common among men than was previously thought. He describes most of this as psychologically based, ranging from the effects of feeling overwhelmed by life events to fears of intimacy.

Women, according to Dr. LoPiccolo, are becoming more likely to question male performance and behavior and are often the ones who will initiate treatment for the male with low sexual interest. But women themselves may exhibit the symptoms. Called by the pejorative term "frigidity," this behavior used to be interpreted as fear and active resistance to sexuality, but now it is more often viewed as low sexual desire and lack of responsiveness.

Although a lack of sexual desire can be a comfortable way of life for some, more often it troubles at least one partner. Sex therapists note that a growing proportion of their patients seek help for what is currently called "inhibited sexual desire." While occasional and short-lived lack of sexual desire is commonplace and reversible, if it is long-lasting, it can be one of the most difficult and intractable of sexual symptoms. For those who wish to change, it is a combination of sex therapy, psychotherapy, and marriage counseling over an extended period of time that may prove to be the most beneficial.

Others experience sexual desire but find that the physical responsiveness is absent. This manifests itself as impotence in men and failure to lubricate and reach orgasm in women. Its causes can encompass a range of emotions from depression, grief, and stress to anxiety, fear, and anger. Ordinarily the sexual response returns when the underlying emotions are resolved or improved. But such psychologically based symptoms, whatever their original emotional cause, can also quickly create performance anxiety and continued sexual problems if people are intimidated, embarrassed, or frightened by the changes in their sexual functioning. This is particularly true of men, for whom "performance" carries great importance.

The first step in self-treatment is for both you and your partner to relax and assume that sexual functioning is likely to improve once emotional equilibrium is restored. Kindness and consideration toward each other and a lack of psychological pressure are crucial for recovery. It is important to remember that a sexual response cannot be willed. It is most likely to occur when a person is rested, relaxed, and in a positive mood, and enjoying a good relationship with his or her partner.

An important way of inducing arousal is through physical stimulation. You should first involve the body as a whole and later focus on the genitals. Masters and Johnson initiated a three-stage method of "sensate focus," which is now used by many sex therapists to teach people to relax and slowly move each other into a state of sexual arousal that eventually results in an orgasm. The stages are, first, to embark step-by-step on a nongenital "pleasuring" of your partner's body by touching and caressing it; second, to touch and caress the genitals, stopping short of actual sex; and third, to engage in nondemanding sexual intercourse where the goal is pleasure rather than performance.

Premature ejaculation also is a fairly common

problem, as it affects 15 to 20 percent of American men, according to Masters and Johnson. While occasional and temporary premature ejaculation happens to most men from time to time (when they have had infrequent sex or are unusually aroused), it usually disappears by itself as circumstances change. However, persistent premature ejaculation is another matter. It does not tend to develop for the first time in the mid or later years but usually begins early on, and it may well continue into later life. Fortunately it is often responsive to treatment. Reassurance is the first step to try, along with making certain there are regular opportunities for sexual outlet.

If these efforts are not enough, a highly successful method has been developed by Masters and Johnson—the "squeeze" technique—in which the woman applies pressure to the head of her partner's erect penis in the following manner: She puts her thumb against the underside of the penis and her index and middle fingers opposite the thumb on either side of the ridge of tissue that separates the head of the penis from the shaft. She then gently presses all three fingers together (her partner can tell her how strongly to squeeze) for a few seconds. This causes the man to lose his urge to ejaculate but allows the couple to continue lovemaking. By alternating the squeezing with sex play, a couple may delay ejaculation until they are ready for a climax. A more detailed description of this technique appears in *Masters and Johnson on Sex and Human Loving* (Little, Brown, 1986).

There is also the "stop-start" technique, which is perhaps the most frequent approach used. It refers to stopping genital stimulation until the urge to ejaculate disappears—at which time stimulation is resumed again. If these techniques fail to work, you may find psychotherapy helpful. In addition, you may find that premature ejaculation may become less of a problem as a man grows older, simply because some of the urgency to ejaculate diminishes.

CHANGES OVER TIME

Role changes over time can also cause disruptions in sexual behavior. One partner may alter his or her level of assertiveness, affecting the original emotional or power balance between the two. We sometimes see relationships in which the man has assumed a predominantly fatherly, protective role toward his more dependent partner. If he becomes sick and needs her care, serious problems, including sexual difficulties, can arise. The woman, who has always been babied, can become petulant, dissatisfied, or simply unable or unwilling to play a giving and responsible role. A variant of this is the hypochondriacal man—the worrywart—involved with an independent and caretaking woman who becomes ill.

When she cannot mother her partner, the equilibrium in which they had functioned for so long is upset as well.

Most typically, women gradually become more assertive and men more nurturant as they grow older. This pattern appears to occur in numerous cultures. One explanation is that it represents a move toward "wholeness" of personality after the cultural and possibly biological emphasis on gender differences in behavior earlier in life, which has young men assuming the assertive roles and young women the nurturing ones.

People may also simply grow tired of their usual roles and desperately desire a change. Sexual boredom and apathy are very common among older couples, who may fall into routine patterns in which they do the same things time after time, year after year, with little imagination in technique or style and a scarcity of zest for creating sexual excitement. Eventually the couple may no longer even care for each other. A new partner may seem to bring improvement, but unless the sources of the underlying boredom are dealt with directly, the improvement may prove only temporary after the novelty has worn off.

Interestingly, relationships that were unstable and unsatisfactory earlier in life sometimes improve in the later years, as the children grow up and leave and the stresses of parenthood and career pass. Personality growth may even lead to greater compatibility. On the other hand, long-standing problems between partners can worsen as the result of chronic irritation from years of unresolved conflict. Personality and behavior changes may also be unilateral: one partner may begin to move in new directions, leaving the other one behind, often angry and hurt.

What should you do if you and your partner are having problems? First, talk to each other about the problems—often. It is important to determine the basis of the problem and then to attempt to resolve it jointly. This, of course, is easier said than done. Be prepared for the fact that each of you may refuse to admit your own contribution to the situation and may place the blame on the other. It is difficult to be open and objective about emotional issues, but it is absolutely essential to realize that what you should be looking for is a *solution* rather than a *culprit*. If you find that you can't get anywhere in trying to talk, go together to your clergyperson, your physician, or a professional psychotherapist or counselor. If your partner won't go, go alone. Late-life separation and/or divorce can be extremely painful and jolting; make the effort to salvage and improve the difficult relationship first. Even if a separation finally occurs, you will be comforted by the notion that you tried, and you will have learned something about yourself and your partner that may help you understand the past and prepare for the future.

LIFE CYCLE CHANGES

DIVORCE

Currently 40 percent of first marriages end in divorce. Of the divorced, 67 percent remarry within five years. And the past five years indicate that we may have stabilized at the current rates of divorce for the present. Some believe that the practical and psychological problems resulting from divorce and remarriage will become so severe that there will be a trend back to preservation of marriages through more skilled premarital and marital counseling (counseling now prevents divorce in only 10 to 15 percent of cases, and conciliations have even less success) and less accessible divorces. Others see the tendency toward remarriages—"serial" marriages—as natural and inevitable as people live longer, divorce is easier to obtain, and women are more independent financially.

This was the case with Patricia, who was finally ready to admit that she wanted a divorce. She had spent forty-five years married to a self-centered, demanding man. Her two sons were in their forties, married and established. Patricia felt she might have a chance to build a new life in her later years. Her husband Herbert was shocked. He couldn't imagine what was wrong. Yet Patricia's desperation and despair were obvious. The two of them were vastly incompatible in personality, interests, and goals. After an effort at marital counseling, they broke up. Herbert never fully understood, but he quickly found another partner and remarried. Patricia relished her new freedom and began to find her own place in the world.

The process of separation and divorce precipitates more couples into professional counseling than any other life crisis, simply because it is so common and so frequently painful. Studies show that, at younger ages, men tend to have greater psychological adjustment problems after divorce than women, although women have far more economic problems, especially if they have children to raise. In the older age groups, the current generation of women appear to have the greater adjustment problems: their financial situation is more precarious, many have no work history outside the home, there are fewer men available for companionship and possible remarriage, and socially, older women alone are often stereotyped as boring and uninteresting. Yet significant numbers of older, divorced women report that they have built interesting and even exciting new lives for themselves.

Separation and divorce can have serious effects on your belief in yourself as a socially and sexually desirable person—particularly if it was your partner who initiated the process. The challenge is to build relationships in which you find support, social approval, friendship, and possibly a new intimacy with another person. We have outlined some suggestions for doing so later in Chapter 7.

YOUNG WIVES/ OLDER HUSBANDS

Younger wives of older husbands frequently express concern about male potency as their husbands reach their sixties. Sometimes the anxiety is unfounded and reassurance is all that is necessary. But there can be real problems and then the young woman's question is "Is there anything that I can do?" The answer is yes, much of which is reviewed in this book. But one point is especially worth emphasizing. Clyde Martin of the Baltimore Longitudinal Study on Aging reports that the capacity of older men for erotic imagery appears somewhat reduced with age. Since so much of sexual desire and performance originates in the mind, this is an important finding. The couple should openly discuss the issue and experiment with increasing their erotic stimuli. What works will be different for each person, whether it involves romantic settings, dancing, erotic films, videos and magazines, music, massage, and the like. Women also need to remember that manual stimulation of their partner's penis is often not only desirable but also necessary after midlife. And finally, reassurance and thoughtfulness on the part of women go a long way in resolving difficulties that may occur as men grow older.

RETIREMENT

Retirement can bring problems as well as possibilities for enhancing relationships. The sudden onset of twenty-four hours a day of togetherness can be a difficult adjustment to make! Such unremitting intimacy places greater pressure on emotional relationships and brings problems into more acute focus, so that what may previously have been an occasional irritant becomes a constant one. A struggle for control over daily activities can become a preoccupation as each partner strives to adjust to the other's frequent presence. Even if you can work out these struggles, the constant togetherness may dismay, disconcert, or irritate you. You must find a balance between shared time and time alone to give each of you elbow room, and you must talk to your partner about your concerns.

Yet retirement has many advantages. Couples have more time to devote to relationships, and many in fact become closer to each other and to other people after retirement. Schedules are also much more flexible, so that one or both members of a couple are less likely to find themselves exhausted when the opportunity for lovemaking arises.

CHRONIC AND INCAPACITATING ILLNESS

Illness may incapacitate one sexual partner physically and/or mentally but not the other, particularly when there is a substantial age gap between them. Frequently the man develops a serious illness first, leaving the woman without a companion or a sexual partner. Healthy women—especially those who are significantly younger than their husbands—may thus spend years in a relationship without adult intimacy or sexual contact. Other feelings can further complicate the picture. When one partner becomes ill, the other ordinarily reacts with concern and the desire to help. But if the illness becomes chronic, the healthy partner may be surprised to find himself or herself filled with anger. This may reflect a defense against the possible loss of the other, but it can also represent overwork, exhaustion, and or an understandable resentment over missing out on life because of the duties of the nursing role and the incapacities of one's partner.

A woman attorney wrote us:

I am a consultant to our local committee on aging and have been asked in private conferences with persons over sixty what the attitude of a spouse should be whose husband/wife is hopelessly ill with dementia in a nursing home. In these cases the future time element is entirely uncertain, but much of the time the patients receive such good care that they may live for years and years and years. Have you written anything on this? Or can you refer me to something that has been written from a realistic viewpoint? I am familiar, of course with the "moralistic" church view that you are married for life. But this is cold comfort to the healthy spouse with a desire to live a full, stimulating, and satisfying life.

It is important that you do not feel guilty about such resentments. Face them frankly and secure outside help whenever possible from your relatives, neighbors, friends, or professional homemakers to reduce your burden. Support groups involving people in similar circumstances can be very helpful. You may recognize that it's necessary to build new friendships to provide a sense of self-worth and companionship.

At other times illness may cause sexual problems, but despite this, you and your partner may still desire and be able to have a relationship that involves closeness and a sense of being valued. A woman tells us that she and her partner are in their seventies. Of her partner she says, "He's never lost his love and tenderness. He's always been a good lover." Yes, they still make love. But they no longer have intercourse because he has prostate cancer.

Again, intercourse is the form of sexual activity that is most likely to be impaired. Both you and your partner may feel guilty, so reassure each other that you can express your sexuality in other satisfying ways. In general, the less goal oriented (in terms of erections and orgasms) and the more flexible you both are, the more likely you both are to develop ways to enjoy lovemaking and each other.

Those with ill or disabled mates at home state that it is difficult to routinely bathe, feed, and provide nursing care for a mate and still think of him or her as sexually desirable. If sexuality is viable and important to you as a couple and you can afford help, hire a visiting nurse or a home-help attendant to take care of the less aesthetic parts of patient care. Returning to your normal roles as closely as possible is the goal. Other ways to adapt positively to the change are to express your feelings to someone you trust, or possibly to your partner; this way you can gather accurate information about your partner's physical problems, become involved in whatever rehabilitation process is feasible, and, if necessary, learn to express caring and sexuality in new ways.

At times a sexual relationship becomes totally untenable. For example, Judy's memory had become increasingly obliterated during the course of Alzheimer's disease. She had always said that she wouldn't want to live if she couldn't have her independence. It had never occurred to her that she might lose her intellectual abilities, her memory, and even her capacity to recognize her loved ones. Her husband, Jim, remained faithful and loving and was her major caregiver. When he would try to feed and dress her, she often became hostile and would even punch him. Jim had long ago lost his sexual desire for her. When he was simply holding her affectionately, she often resisted him or would even push him away. At other times she seemed aroused and would press him sexually, and he found it difficult to respond. Jim found relief by joining a group of caregivers with similar problems. He quickly learned to accept his reactions without feeling guilty or disloyal to the memory of his long and mostly happy relationship.

As strange as it might seem, the knowledge that an illness of one partner may be terminal or fatal sometimes brings an improvement or a heightening of a relationship. Couples report that the certainty or closeness of death causes them to cherish the present and to take advantage of the time they have left together. When sexuality is a part of that closeness, such couples should always have the opportunity for privacy and time alone, even if one partner is confined to a hospital or another institution. If you encounter problems in working this out with an institution, discuss the situation with a patient representative or a social worker on staff.

INSTITUTIONAL LIVING

The 5 percent of persons over sixty-five who live in homes for the aging, nursing homes, chronic-disease hospitals, and other long-term-care institutions are in general denied the opportunity for any private social and sexual life. Visitors are often in full view of roommates and staff and can easily be overheard by them. Even those who have marital partners are seldom able to share conjugal visits, as they usually are not afforded a private time and place with their partners.

As to unmarried people who reside in nursing homes, intimacies of any kind—even hugging, kissing, or holding hands—may be frowned on despite the fact that they are performed by consenting adults. Even those who understandably resort to self-stimulation because they have no other sexual outlet run the risk of being discovered and reprimanded like children.

Most older persons living under these conditions are reluctant to complain to the management, even though their rights as adults are being seriously infringed on. Ask the administrator of your particular institution to provide whatever privacy you and other patients should have. If you need outside support, ask your relatives, friends, doctor, lawyer, or a member of the clergy to help you in stating your case. Speak to others who have a similar complaint and make it a joint project.

If this fails, alert groups that are interested in the problems of older persons, such as local chapters of the Gray Panthers, the Older Women's League, the American Association of Retired Persons, and the National Council of Senior Citizens. Federal regulations issued on June 1, 1978, provide some right to privacy, but only for married couples, and only in nursing homes that participate in federal Medicare and Medicaid programs (more than two-thirds do not). These regulations are not being uniformly enforced, but failure to observe them *is* ground for legal action. For detailed information, write Health Standards and Quality Bureau, Office of Standards and Certification, Health Care Financing Administration, 6325 Security Blvd., Baltimore, Maryland 21207.

WIDOWHOOD

Unfortunately, the possibility of widowhood increases with age. Losses and grieving are inevitable as we grow older, and need to be worked through and accepted, so that the survivor may resume a full life or shape a new and different one. Losing someone you have loved— partner, friend, child—usually means shock and then a long, slow journey through grief. Acute grief, with the attendant mental anguish and remorse, ordinarily lasts a month or two and then begins to lessen. In most cases, grief works itself out in six to eighteen months unless it is complicated by further loss, stress, or other factors. *Widow shock,* an exaggerated state that can follow the sudden and unexpected death of a partner, or occurs when the surviving partner is ill-prepared to handle living alone, leaves the survivor unable to accept death and take up life again. To recover, he or she needs to be encouraged to grieve and should be assisted in building an active life once more. The open expression of feelings, including crying, is important for both men and women in resolving their grief. Sharing your sadness, anger, resentment, fear, and self-pity with someone else helps.

Such *grief work* also involves talking about your sexual feelings. A newly widowed woman says of her sexuality:

> My husband died eight months ago. I would like some information about what happens to widows like me. I am surprised to find that one of the things I miss the most is my sex life. I feel so empty and alone now.

People need to separate out their own identities from the commingling of identities that has occurred in close and long-term relationships. The feeling that "part of me died with him [her]" can then be replaced with the feeling that "I am a person in myself and I am still alive." A man may find himself temporarily impotent, a symptom we call widower's syndrome; this usually clears up if he is encouraged to grieve and find his way through the loss.

Anticipatory grief, during which a person undergoes an extended grief reaction prior to the expected death of the loved one—as happens in the course of a terminal illness—can soften the shock of death. Although such grieving may result in a closer relationship with the ill partner, there are instances when the grieving person may close himself or herself off, as though the partner were already dead. If this occurs, you need outside counseling to reestablish the relationship with the dying person.

After the death of a partner, the man or woman who has been widowed may find it hard to look ahead to a new partner without feelings of guilt or disloyalty. In *enshrinement,* the survivor keeps things just as they were when the loved one was alive and spends his or her energy revering the memory of the dead person. The survivor believes that to live fully is a betrayal of love or loyalty for the dead. This survival guilt and fear of infidelity leads to emotional stagnation and stands in the way of achieving new relationships. Once the period of mourning is over and the initial shock and grief have abated, *you owe it to yourself* to become realistic about your need to have a new life of your own. This means you should preserve your memories appropriately, without excessive dwelling in the past. Jim, who is eighty-one, described his complicated feelings: "I took care of Flo through the awful time—the diagnosis of her cancer, the chemotherapy, the radiation; it was miserable. She could not eat; for that matter, I couldn't either. We would hold each other, but that was about all. After a while, I have to say that it was not very pleasant even to touch her. It was awful. I felt guilty about that. After she died, I grieved for a long time. I didn't think that I would want to have anything to do with anybody.

"But about three months ago I met Marjorie at a school function for my grandson. She was a widow, too. She had lost her husband even before Flo died. It was like starting all over again. I was like a schoolboy. It took me some nerve to ask her to have lunch, but we did. We have gotten together a lot—to movies and dinner and various places—and I have held her hand and kissed her. But I feel guilty and disloyal to Flo."

In a support group designed for newly widowed persons, Jim learned that what he had been going through was *widower's guilt*, a common reaction in which the memory of one's dead partner becomes a roadblock to taking up life again. Jim participated enthusiastically in the group, and as the weeks went by, he began to build new relationships, including a compatible one with Marjorie.

The usual cure for both widower's guilt and enshrinement is to take an active role in getting life moving again. This is an act of will and determination. It can happen *only* if the individual decides to make it happen. You should remove from sight the personal possessions of the deceased, and put away such obvious marriage symbols as the wedding ring. It is *not* a betrayal of a past marriage to accept the present and build a future.

If your grief and anger over a death continue unchanged for years, then there is something interfering with the natural healing process of time. Quite often it is unresolved negative feelings toward the dead person (as in an unhappy marriage) or a stubborn refusal to accept fate and take positive steps toward creating a new life. In these cases, seek professional counseling.

For those aged fifty-five or older, the American Association of Retired Persons has a Widowed Persons Service in some 240 locations nationwide. A volunteer who has gone through the same experience will talk to the newly widowed person about his or her feelings, and help with any problems (write to: AARP, 601 E Street, N.W., Washington, DC 20049).

Remember, it *is* possible to develop a new, exciting and fulfilling life for yourself even *after* the death of your partner. A seventy-six-year-old widow recently let us know that:

> I find myself in love with a wonderful gentleman of eighty-three years whom I met about six weeks ago after two months of letter writing. (He saw an advertisement I placed in the *Jewish Monthly,* looking for someone to correspond with.)
>
> I recently felt the need to write a poem about how I felt. Here it is:

Widow's Love in Spring

> Love in the Spring,
> Can't do any old thing,
> Just thinking of my Love

All day long.
Waiting to see him and feel his
Arms around me,
Wanting his lips on mine,
So tender and sweet.
Oh, the life of a widow
So happy and free
All because of
Love in the Spring.

CHAPTER 7

❦

FINDING
NEW RELATIONSHIPS

THE DEMOGRAPHIC
DILEMMA

As they grow older, many people find themselves without partners. This is especially true of women because of their longer life expectancies and lower rates of remarriage after widowhood. Until medical science and public health programs (such as prevention of late-life illness, disability, and, for many men, early death) become more successful in equalizing the life expectancies of men and women, we shall have to tolerate the social consequences of greater numbers of single women over sixty than single men. However, women are adapting in a number of ways: by challenging negative cultural stereotypes of them, both personally and institutionally through organizations such as the Older Women's League and the Gray Panthers; by learning to take the initiative in building friendships and a social life; and by redefining their own sexuality to include a wider range of options for satisfying intimacy and sexual release. Some are developing relationships with younger men. Others have relationships with married men who may be unable or unwilling to leave their marriages. Some sublimate their sexuality by developing absorbing activities that bring them companionship and accomplishment. Lesbian women are in a particularly advantageous position as they reach midlife and beyond, since partners who are their own age will have a similar life expectancy, and they move in a world that becomes increasingly female with each decade.

None of this, however, negates the necessity of searching for ways to increase the life expectancy of men as well as preserving their physical vigor and sexual functioning as they grow older. Fortunately, we are already seeing improvements. There has been a dramatic drop in deaths from heart disease since the early 1970s for both black and white males, and more recently, a drop in lung cancer death rates for white males.

Yet the likelihood of losing your partner is a fact of late life that increases with time. In 1992 over 48 percent of all women sixty-five and over were widowed. Only 15 percent of men 65 and over were widowed. Another 5 percent of men and women this age had never married, and about 4 percent were divorced. Obviously there are differences between the life-style of those who never married and who over the years have created a circle of friends and intimates that substitutes for an immediate family, and those who are abruptly separated from a spouse by death or divorce and now find themselves on their own for the first time in many years or possibly in their lives. Where the widowed person is deprived of the shared intimacies and interdependence of long marriage and the social patterns that go with being a couple, the single or long-divorced man or woman is accustomed to living on his or her own. Still, as one grows older, time and deaths among one's peers erode the circle of relatives and close friends regardless of marital status. This can lead to an increasing emptiness in the later years that needs to be filled with new relationships.

BUILDING A
NEW SOCIAL LIFE

You cannot depend on the healing power of time alone to ease grief or loss or to alleviate loneliness. New relationships will not simply happen. You will have to take an active part in putting your life together again. Molly, age seventy-eight, and her late husband, Frank, had discussed their feelings long before he died. They had agreed that life should go on after one of them died, and that the survivor should feel free to explore new relationships and build a new life. This is exactly what Molly did. She became attracted to Ben, but decided to take her time before getting heavily involved with anyone. She did not want to rush into anything; it was time for her to enjoy her new life of dating and exploration.

WHERE DO YOU START?

Take the initiative. It is up to you to take charge of your life, to decide what you want and what you should do about it. This does not mean you must be searching for a possible partner. You may want no more than opportunities to meet people who are congenial and likely to share your own interests. One way to do this is to look for activities that support these interests. You will feel less tense and pressured if you are doing what you like to do. A sense of pleasure and purpose in what you are doing will encourage you to enjoy, learn, give of yourself, and make friends.

SOME PEOPLE WORRY ABOUT ETIQUETTE

Many older people are still bound by the customs they were taught as youngsters, yet many of these formalities make no sense today. Women used to be told it was improper to call a man. But if you are interested, you do *not* have to wait for invitations from a man; simply behave as you do when you want to get in touch with a friend. He has the option of accepting or refusing, just as you do when a man (or woman) calls you. If he accepts your invitation, a friendship or a relationship may develop or it may not—but you will have taken a perfectly appropriate and dignified initiative that allows you an *active* role in finding new friends and activities.

WHAT ACTIVITIES SHOULD YOU TRY?

A variety of activities are available to older, single people who want to develop a fuller social life. Among the best opportunities are those afforded through work. If you do not have a job but are interested and able, consider the possibility of looking actively for part-time work, both for the rewards of being useful and for the opportunities it offers to meet new people under daily and unselfconscious circumstances.

Where you live will affect the number of choices you have for activities that will widen your social circle. Except in isolated rural communities there are more possibilities than you may realize. If you are politically minded, for example, you can volunteer to help at your local political club. Volunteer work for worthwhile causes, social service agencies, or nearby hospitals or schools may provide you with personal rewards at the same time that it brings you into contact with other people who share similar concerns. Those who like to be active and out-of-doors can seek out health clubs, hiking and biking clubs, wilderness, nature, and birdwatching groups.

If you can't find something that fits your particular taste, consider organizing it yourself. Any special interests can lead to social contacts. Musicians can start amateur chamber music groups, orchestras, or jazz, western, country, and ethnic music groups. Many towns and cities have amateur choirs, where an interest in singing is the only prerequisite. Painting, theater, handicraft, and folk art clubs are popular; if there is a Y in your community, you may find it is already sponsoring such activities. One midwestern woman started a sewing circle aimed specifically at men who wanted to learn how to quilt and do needlepoint. Organizing potluck dinners is a good way to cut costs and promote sociability. Cooking clubs are popular among both men and women. Woodworking and carpentry, wine making and tasting, chess and investment clubs, and bridge and other card and game clubs can be comfortable ways to meet people.

If you live in a city or its suburbs, you have the advantage of a wider choice of activities. Senior centers and community centers offer recreational opportunities; there are now at least ten thousand senior centers and clubs in the United States, operated by churches, synagogues, social clubs, and nonprofit corporations. These centers offer shows, parties, music, beauty salons, handicrafts, trips, discussion groups, and a variety of other things to do at the same time you are encountering new people.

Religious activities are another important way of meeting people. Many churches and synagogues sponsor singles clubs, and some are beginning to expand these to fit the needs of people in the mid and later years. Talk to your local cleric about starting such a group if one does not exist in your locale. If you are the parent of a child or an adolescent, Parents Without Partners clubs can be a source of contacts and of help to you, both as a parent and as a single person.

If you live in a rural area or a small town, you are more likely to know everyone who might be available as a friend or a companion in your area, just as they, in turn, know you. For variety you may want to make and visit friends in neighboring communities and get to larger urban areas for activities whenever possible. Trips and vacations away from home can be a way of making new acquaintances. If you don't have a car, arrange to share rides with others if you can. Neighbors and friends may be willing to serve as a taxi for you, or you may be able to go by bus.

A small but growing number of older people have begun to live together in communal settings as a means of increasing their social contacts, cutting costs, and sharing housekeeping duties. Some communes are made up only of older people, while others include people of all ages. Most of these are in large houses, although we have also heard of large apartments that are occupied communally and are free of the chores of caring for a house and yard.

The two major organizations for older people, the National Council of Senior Citizens (national office at 1331 F Street, N.W., Washington, DC 20004) and the American Association of Retired Persons—National Retired Teachers Association (national office at 1909 K Street, N.W., Washington, DC 20049), may have chapters in your area where meetings of many kinds take place. Look in your phone book, or if necessary, check with their national offices to see if there is a chapter near you. The AARP alone has thirty-two million members, which provides for significant political advocacy and services (such as discount drugs, insurance coverage supplemental to Medicare, low-cost travel) as well as social opportunities. Widowed older people have been finding support and direction for their lives through the Widow to Widow program, which originated in Boston and is now being sponsored in other cities by the AARP.

If you would like to combine opportunities for meeting people with social and political activism, the Gray Panthers (311 South Juniper Street, Philadelphia, PA 19107), which works vigorously on behalf of the older population, is adding local chapters rapidly, and includes younger as well as older people in its membership. The National Caucus on the Black Aged (2801 14th Street, N.W., 1st Floor, Washington, DC 20009) focuses specifically on the problems of older African-American people.

Ocean cruises can be fun, and some people do meet partners this way, although the cruises generally attract more women than men and are expensive. If you have the money, are interested in where you are going, and like to travel, you can enjoy yourself and make friends on a cruise. Don't be afraid to ask the ship's purser for help in meeting others and seating you with compatible dining companions. Younger men who are attracted to older women may use cruises as a meeting place; be careful that they aren't interested chiefly in your money.

A more inexpensive way to travel sociably is to go on bus tours, some of which cover the entire United States and parts of Canada. You can get a ticket for use nationwide at reasonable rates. Take a friend, go by yourself or with a group, and be open to meeting new people along the way.

The travel industry is actively promoting travel for

single people of all ages, with special seminars, tips for solo travelers, and tour packages. Club Med (800-258-2633), the Sierra Club trips (718-370-2096), Smithsonian Associate tours (202-357-2888 for overseas tours), Lindblad Travel vacations (booked through travel agents), and Elderhostel programs (100 Boylston Street, Suite 200, Boston, Massachusetts 02160, and 55 Chapel Street, Newton, Massachusetts 02160) are popular with single people. Singleworld (booked through travel agents) offers worldwide cruises and tours for those traveling alone. Travel Companion Exchange (516-454-0880) uses computerized listings to help pair single people together for all sorts of travel—not just to arrange companions but to avoid the penalty many hotels, tours, and cruises place on single travelers.

Dance lessons are widely touted for older people, but be wary: the commercial ones can be greatly overpriced and sometimes fraudulent, offering "lifetime contracts" and noncancelable contracts. If you can't locate a reputable and reasonably priced place to learn, find friends who will teach you. If you are a good dancer, offer to teach someone else. Square dancing, folk dancing, and ballroom dancing may bring back memories (as well as the dance steps themselves!) from your past. A number of cities have relatively inexpensive public ballrooms; Roseland in New York, for example, has ballroom dancing (predominantly frequented by the elderly) on Thursdays and Sundays. Friendships and romances can begin in such settings—Roseland has a plaque on its wall engraved with the names of married couples who first met there.

High school, college, and other reunions offer men and women the chance to renew acquaintance with compatible people they knew earlier in life, who are now widowed or divorced themselves. So go to them! It is not uncommon for childhood sweethearts to meet again and even marry after each has raised a family and been widowed. Family reunions and family contacts in general are another way to get in touch with people who may be seeking new relationships; there is a long and honorable tradition, for example, of widows and widowers who are in-laws developing close relationships that end in marriage or partnership.

Commercial singles clubs and computer dating services are growing in popularity, especially for the young and middle-aged. But there is no reason why older people can't use them as well. Personal ads, too, have become popular and even reputable. For a small fee you can dream up a description of yourself and the kind of partner you are looking for and place it in the classified section of a wide variety of newspapers and magazines. Your identity is protected by a post office box number unless and until you choose to reveal yourself to a respondent.

If you are simply looking for an escort or temporary companion for a business or social event, there are legitimate agencies that will provide people, for a fee. Some escort services, however, are fronts for hiring sex partners (both male and female). If you are uneasy about commercial escort services, ask your local cleric whether he or she knows someone who could accompany you, or get in touch with an older persons' group or senior center.

Don't overlook born matchmakers among your friends, acquaintances, colleagues, children, or other family members. Some people have highly developed sensibilities and can be very helpful in finding men or women you would enjoy meeting. But save yourself time and trouble by picking your matchmaker carefully; look for someone whose judgment you respect and who knows you well.

QUALITIES THAT FOSTER NEW RELATIONSHIPS

When you first venture to meet new people, it will help to remember that they are as likely to be feeling as tentative or shy as you. And what you look for in other people—companionship, friendship, relationships— are usually the same types of things they are seeking from you. When you do strike up an acquaintance, be warm and sensitive to the other person's feelings. It doesn't matter if you are quiet or lively—everyone's temperament is different—but in either case, it is well regarded if you display curiosity and an active mind. People also appreciate imagination, responsiveness, and a sense of humor.

That said, there are certain personal qualities that foster the art of making friends. Most people respond to a sense of vitality and energy. Those who are pleasantly assertive (not domineering) have a greater chance of meeting new people and forming rewarding relationships—and it's simply because they do not leave all the initiative up to others.

QUALITIES THAT HINDER NEW RELATIONSHIPS

It is important to maintain a positive approach, one that transcends or tempers any problems you have. Many older people have endured the deaths of spouses or friends, difficulties with children, financial burdens, loneliness, and an increasing feeling of uselessness. Under these pressures, it is not uncommon for you to feel that life has been unfair and to bear a grudge against your circumstances. But this resentment is likely to make other people wary of becoming involved with you. It is depressing to be with someone who is complaining or petulant and whose outlook is pessimistic. So make a deliberate, conscious act of will to overcome the perception that all seems sour in your life. If you don't do this, you'll be hindering your chances for new and enriching relationships.

CAN YOU BE EXPLOITED?

When someone "uses" someone else in an emotional relationship without giving much in return, it's exploitation. It is up to you—and only you!—to know what to look out for and how to protect yourself. Some older men (and, far more rarely, women) marry primarily to gain a housekeeper or nurse. Well, the "romance" is going to disappear as soon as the marriage vows are exchanged and the woman discovers she has been recruited primarily to perform these services. It is much wiser, of course, to take the time to learn as much as you can about the other person before you decide to marry. The history of his or her relationships with the opposite sex can be incredibly illuminating. Most exploiters have a long history of taking advantage of others.

In other instances the exploiter may primarily be after your money or property. Matrimonial swindles through lonely-hearts clubs and correspondence with strangers who claim a romantic interest in you are notorious. The tip-off comes when the person begins to be inordinately interested in your property, your money, or your will. *If you suspect this is happening to you, get to a lawyer, cleric, or someone else you can trust, and ask for advice.*

SPECIAL PROBLEMS FOR WOMEN

Unattached older women, especially those who are widowed or divorced, often find themselves left out of activities that involve couples. Hostesses at dinner parties feel they must have a man available for each woman guest, with couples coming two by two like the creatures on Noah's Ark. The hostess may also find the presence of a widow or divorcee uncomfortable because she fears possible competition.

If you are frequently left out socially, one solution is to join with other single people and organize your own activities. Or develop a circle of friends in which friendship rather than gender is the key to getting together, and where people of any age, sex, or marital status can enjoy one another's company. Start inviting your own married friends along; in the process they may become less inflexible about their own social habits in inviting guests!

If you are divorced, be prepared to have some people see you as a failure. Others can make the conscious or unconscious assumption that the breakup of your marriage was caused by a flaw in you. Get support by talking this over with understanding people who care about you.

Both widows and divorcees find that some men (married or otherwise) assume that women who are sexually experienced are automatically available and willing. Indeed, these men may see themselves as doing you a sexual favor. If this expectation annoys or upsets you, tell them so. If they don't understand, write off the relationship.

Single women who have never married have their own set of concerns:

> Your book *Love and Sex After Sixty* is fine for married couples, but what about a single person who has never had sex? Naturally, I have always been curious, but I would be terrified to indulge. I never had a date until I was thirty, and every man I went on a date with expected sex in return. Out of fear, I stopped dating. Sex is for *after* marriage. Of course, I blame myself for not being married, and you can't blame a man for trying. But the man who is looking for a wife doesn't want someone already picked over, so I've remained single and lonely.

If this situation is yours, we recommend that you speak to a professional counselor who should be able to help allay many of your concerns. And there *are* men out there who are not looking for immediate sexual involvement.

SPECIAL PROBLEMS FOR MEN

As a general rule, unattached men have fewer *social* difficulties. Even those who had not thought themselves socially very accomplished when they were younger may be surprised to find how eagerly accepted and actively pursued they now are. (This is largely because there are fewer men than women.) One eighty-one-year-old man told us:

> I have scarcely had a moment alone since my wife died of a long illness last year. The ladies in my church have taken pity on me as "a helpless man," I guess. I had more food appearing at my front door than you could imagine—it was a regular casserole brigade for weeks after my wife died! I was in too much shock and upset at the time to see all the humor in this. But we men are in big demand in old age. I for one think it's great!

So if you are a man who enjoys relationships with women, you are likely to have ample opportunity for them! On the other hand, if you are a man who finds it annoying or troubling to be treated like a commodity in short supply, you will have to make this clear or else remove yourself from those situations where this tends to occur.

Uncertainty can be a problem for men. Many men,

like many women, are hesitant, shy, or dubious about their ability to handle personal relationships. To find yourself valued as an available man as you grow older is not automatically reassuring if you doubt your sophistication, skill, or appeal to the opposite sex. Most men have been conditioned to believe that anything short of total self-confidence is shameful, a failure of "masculinity." Though a woman may have similar problems of self-confidence, society has not pressured her into feeling "unwomanly" as a result. If you are troubled by doubts about your skill in social and sexual situations, recognize that you have plenty of company, and that this insecurity reflects in no way on your degree of manliness. Most women you meet are not going to measure you against some impossible ideal and judge you a failure. Further, the man who is shy, diffident, or uncertain about his competence will have to make the same effort of will, and exercise the same degree of initiative, that a hesitant woman must undertake. You will discover if you do not take this step that relationships are no more likely to happen for you than they would for her.

SPECIAL PROBLEMS FOR LESBIAN AND GAY RELATIONSHIPS

It has long been a common belief that life becomes increasingly bleak and lonely as the lesbian or gay man grows older. This is by no means inevitably true. An estimated 10 percent or more of all Americans are ho-mosexual; and, similar to the heterosexual population, many gay men and women have long-term relation-ships, are emotionally stable, and are successful and happy even in their later years.

When difficulties, both social and sexual, occur for lesbian or gay male couples, they involve many of the same interpersonal problems faced by heterosexual cou-ples. But in addition, lesbian and gay couples may find themselves isolated in the larger society, with too few role models for growing older as members of a gay part-nership or as single people. There can be a lack of sup-port from friends, relatives and others when a longtime companion is ill or dies. Often hospitals and other insti-tutions do not recognize the gay relationship in terms of visitation rights and consultation with medical person-nel. Legal rights are often unclear and unprotected; for example, relatives of the deceased can and do contest wills if belongings are left to the deceased's unmarried partner.

The current generation of lesbian and gay elders grew up in a difficult era of change and challenge. Before the turn of the century, few homosexuals in the United States had any sense of community with others like themselves, or any feeling of acceptance in the larger world. Most married and either lived double lives or suppressed their sexual inclinations. The earlier part of the century brought greater freedom, especially for those in large urban areas. But it was not until the late

1960s, when the modern gay liberation movement began, that the homosexual community forged a real sense of solidarity and won greater social acceptance. Thus many older lesbians and gay men have gone through major struggles both personally and socially. A goodly number are still in the closet, living as "roommates," "sisters," "brothers," and so on. All face the tremendously complicated new challenge of the AIDS crisis, which has drawn both attention and resources away from other issues of aging in the gay community (see the section on AIDS on pages 77–84).

Nonetheless, organizations *are* beginning to form to aid lesbians and gay men as they reach their later years. SAGE (Senior Action in the Gay Environment) at 208 West 13th Street, New York, New York 10011 offers a variety of social services to older members in the New York metropolitan area and promotes the opportunity for intergenerational support. Write to them for their newsletter *Voices* or call them at 212-721-2247. The National Association of Lesbian and Gay Gerontologists is actively promoting understanding and service for the homosexual community in mid and later life. It offers a quarterly newsletter, *Making a Difference,* and has compiled *Resource Guide: Lesbian and Gay Aging*; both can be obtained by writing to The National Association of Lesbian and Gay Gerontologists, 1853 Market Street, San Francisco, California 94103.

Those located near Washington, D.C., can contact GLOW (Gay and Lesbian Older Washingtonians), P.O.

Box 75195, Washington, DC 20013, at 301-857-3966. This organization provides education services on aging and offers a Drop-in Center Thursday and Saturday at The Gay Community Center of Washington, DC. GLOE (Operation Concern—Gay and Lesbian Outreach to Elders), 1853 Market Street, San Francisco, California 94103, at 415-626-7000, offers a monthly newsletter *GLOE Outreach to Elders* and provides services to gay men and lesbians sixty years and older. They offer information, referral, counseling, support groups, a legal clinic, education forums, and special events. Lesbian women should write for *Golden Threads*, P.O. Box 3177, Burlington, Vermont 05401, a publication for lesbians over fifty and those involved with them, with the purpose of making it possible, in a caring and confidential way, for lesbians to develop friendships even when they are socially isolated. This quarterly publication has an international circulation and contains editorials and book reviews slanted toward the interests of older lesbians; it also includes a large resource list. DIGNITY/USA Task Force on Aging, at 235 South 23rd Street, #3R, Philadelphia, Pennsylvania 19103, or 215-732-3831, studies aging nationwide. It is developing a network of chapters nationwide and with other organizations concerned with older lesbians and gay men. It publishes a nationwide directory of organizations/services for older lesbians/gay men and has developed a resource packet for workshops. Also, *The Legal Guide for Lesbian and Gay Couples* by Hayden Curry and Denis

Clifford (Nolo Press, 1986) covers important legal and financial aspects of lesbian and gay relationships.

It is important to note that research in the gay community is moving away from a global perspective on homosexuality and is concentrating more specifically on aspects of aging. Examples are research directed at the gay male or lesbian couple aging together; the "gay widow"; married or bisexual gay/lesbian aging; the single older gay/lesbian; aged gay men and lesbians in the gay community; special therapy and counseling needs of the older lesbian and gay men; and adult children of gay men and lesbians. Please also refer to the Bibliography, which lists a number of titles of special interest to older gay men and lesbians.

As a Relationship Develops

New anxieties may occur as a relationship progresses to sexual involvement. When men or women doubt their sexual performance, or fear that the person with whom they are involved may be measuring them against the behavior of a previous partner, it will affect their sexual ability. It takes an active effort by both you and your current partner to make the present moment satisfying.

Do not allow memories of past lovemaking to dominate the present. What each of you can give the other should concern you more than anything else, and especially more than anything that was in the past. If a caring person offers reassurance to a partner who is feeling uncertain about his or her skill, it will help restore confidence. Yes, deeply rooted sexual problems may require professional help, but the self-doubt that has its roots in shyness and uneasiness about performance—which is much more common—is often alleviated by thoughtfulness and tenderness.

HANDLING REFUSALS, REBUFFS, AND DISAPPOINTMENTS

However confident they may appear on the surface, a great many men and women worry about rebuffs when they initiate or respond to a social opportunity. How can you best handle such refusals and disappointments? It *is* natural to feel hurt, but you should not let this feeling persist. You have to face the possibility of rejection whenever you involve yourself with others, so be matter-of-fact about it. It is, after all, the other person's right— as it is yours when you are approached. It should not deter you from further involvements. Rejection is nature's way of keeping two people apart who should not be together.

Obviously, there will be some occasions when a person rudely rejects you and doesn't take into account your feelings. These times will be unpleasant and sometimes painful. Unfortunately, this is an unavoidable aspect of human relationships. The point to remember is that *refusals or disappointment do not mean you are a failure as a person.* If you are losing confidence and feel you need a fresh perspective on yourself, talk over your experiences with a close friend. Then draw on the experience you have gained and try again. Take a few chances. Above all, do not waste time berating yourself for what does not work out. Not everything is your responsibility; some aspects of relationships are out of your control.

MOVING TOO FAST

What if one partner in a newly acquainted couple moves too quickly toward intimacy? There is always the widow who is husband-hunting or the man who is on the make sexually on the first date. Carla, age eighty-eight, had met the latter:

> I liked Max immediately when I first met him. (He's eighty-four.) But he was too fast for me: He just barged ahead without looking for any signals. He seemed hell-bent on sex. Now that I think about it, he has had three marriages and two of them have been di-

vorces. He probably has made a habit of demanding his own way. Maybe I'll tell him what I think. What have I got to lose?

Use your common sense and don't be afraid to tell the other person if you are feeling pushed. You have the right to have your feelings respected. If you are one of those impulsive or action-oriented individuals, be sensitive to your companions's feelings. A relationship that is going to be more than merely temporary needs time to build. Explore each other's feelings and learn more about each other. Decide *together* what pace to set. Many people are not ready for physical intimacies— much less marriage—until they feel a mutual understanding and affection. An enduring partnership is based on thoughtfulness as well as attraction. If he or she is not willing to provide you with the time that you need, it may simply mean that there is someone else out there more suited to your temperament.

ARRANGING FOR PRIVACY WHEN YOU LIVE WITH YOUR CHILDREN

Living with your children—as roughly 20 percent of older people do—can certainly put a damper on your social life unless you take preventive steps. And don't depend on your children to recognize your needs for privacy. You will need to take the initiative and discuss this with them frankly. Work out ways of sharing the space in the home, so that there will be times when you can entertain people privately. Some houses are large enough for you to have your own suite of rooms, which makes a separate social life easier. But most older people will have a bedroom at most, and sometimes even this will have to be shared with another member of the family. If you have your own room and it is a reasonable size, you can furnish it as a combination bedroom–sitting room and entertain your friends there. If small children live in the house, put a lock or latch on the door to keep them from running in and out until they learn to knock and enter only on invitation. Your bed can be a couch by day, and you should also have a comfortable chair and other amenities for entertaining. If you must share a bedroom, arrange to have sole use of the room at certain times. There may be difficulties in entertaining privately in the family living or dining room unless you and your family have worked out a practical schedule. It is easier if there is also a recreation room or den. If your resources permit, finance the construction of additional space or undertake some remodeling to gain desired privacy.

It is extremely important that you make your children aware of your desire for privacy *before* you move in with them. Discussing the issue before actual situations arise is more likely to produce results. When it is they who are moving in with you, things are usually a bit easier because you are on your own territory to begin with. The crucial element in living successfully with your children in their home is to be able to talk openly with them about problems and cooperate in solving them.

UNMARRIED AND LIVING TOGETHER

Many couples who come to care for each other want to marry; for them marriage confirms the permanence and depth of their commitment. In addition, for some older people the idea of living together without marriage goes against their moral or religious scruples. But the number of unmarried men and women of all ages living together as sexual partners has increased from two million in 1984 to nearly three million in 1990. Little is known about the myriad reasons unmarried older persons live together. The decision a couple makes may involve deliberate choice, but it also may be the result of necessity. Two people may care deeply for each other but feel that marriage would set limits on an independence they have come to value. Many older men and women who nursed partners through a long chronic illness until death may now feel they do not want to enter into another marriage that might put them through that same ordeal all over again.

There are also instances in which marriage is not an option, and people embark on affairs. Everyone knows of unhappy marriages that continue for years because one partner will not agree to divorce, in effect forcing the other to seek a partner outside marriage. In other marriages, one member may have been incapacitated or chronically ill for a long time, leaving the other without a satisfying sexual and emotional outlet. Affairs are more likely to occur if the marital couple had an unsatisfying emotional relationship to begin with, or if one partner is mentally impaired or institutionalized.

Sometimes the children of a widowed parent object strongly to his or her dating or remarriage. This may cause the parent to avoid relationships because of the fear of family conflict. If this happens, you owe it to yourself to initiate discussions with your children to resolve your differences. If all else fails, call in an outside and objective mediator.

Economic factors may also enter into decisions not to remarry. While recent legislation has improved this situation, there may be pension penalties in cases of remarriage. State Medicaid benefits can also be a barrier. If one partner has been receiving Medicaid, marriage would mean suspending that support until at least a major portion of the savings of the new spouse was used up; only then could Medicaid be resumed. Indeed, there have been cases where husband and wife divorced each other, but continued to live together in order for one of them to be eligible for Medicaid.

In general, the decision of whether to marry or to live together is a private one, to be reached by each individual couple. A host of influences can impact their decision, including religious attitudes, the reactions of relatives, financial considerations, and personal preferences. Everyone should go with the solution that best suits their individual circumstances.

CHAPTER 8

❧❧

LEARNING NEW
PATTERNS OF
LOVEMAKING

If you have been thinking about some aspects of your sex life that you would like to alter, *now* is the time to do it. Don't believe people who tell you that as you grow older you become too fixed in your ways to change. If you were always interested in learning and changing in your past, that attitude is likely to remain with you all your life. Besides which, scientific studies have proved beyond question that older people can learn as well as, and in some cases better than, the young.

Nevertheless, be careful not to underestimate the strength of habit, which can be even greater when it's unconscious; lovemaking patterns tend to become fixed and uninspired over the years, often because you have neither taken the time nor thought it necessary to examine them. Well, it's now time to look with a critical eye at how you have been handling sexual intimacy. Do you always make love at the same time of day and in the same manner? Are you excited and interested in your love life? Do you and your partner know how to please each other? It may be time to loosen up and try something new. Learn to relish once again the special warmth and intimacy that are possible through love and sex.

THE SETTING FOR SEX

Look at your bedroom with a critical eye. Is it comfortable and pleasant? Is it a good place for sex? A firm, comfortable bed for two should be standard equipment unless illness, sleeping problems, or personal preference lead you to choose single beds. In this case the best arrangement is one double bed for making love, talking, and so on, with a single bed in the same room or another room when you are ready to separate for sleep. A double bed encourages the closeness and sharing that enrich a couple's sense of togetherness.

Many older people develop the habit of lining up their medications on their bed stands. This is both aesthetically unattractive and dangerous. When you are drowsy you may fail to read the labels, take the wrong pills in the middle of the night, or accidentally take too many. So place all medications out of sight, at a walking distance from the bed unless they are absolutely essential for emergencies (for example, nitroglycerin for those with heart problems). In addition to protecting yourself, you will not be continually confronting yourself and your partner with reminders of your pains or infirmities.

Another thing that has struck us about many older people's bedrooms is the gallery of family pictures—children, grandchildren, nephews, nieces, and ancestors—that often lines the walls. This is fine for a couple married for many years, who feels comfortable in this setting, but it can be quite unnerving, to say the least, for a new partner, who settles down expectantly in the bed only to find your relatives looking down on the proceedings. Be sensitive to your new partner's feelings. If family pictures are interfering with your love life, banish them to another room.

THE TIME FOR SEX

Finding the best time for sexual activity can greatly enhance a sexual relationship. Having sex exclusively at bedtime is an easy habit to get into over the years, especially if daytime privacy is hard to come by and the pressures of work and family crowd your days. Yet this may not really be your favorite time, and if you are over sixty, it may not be your most energetic period either. For those who are overstressed, overworked, and want or need to make love at night, set aside several evenings a week, relax, and go to bed early, before exhaustion sets in. As to other favorable times for lovemaking: Some couples sleep first and make love in the morning. Others wake each other in the middle of the night, when both have had some rest. Many men report greater sexual potency after a good night's sleep. The morning is a favorite time for many older people because they are rested and relaxed. Daytime naps when possible can make for greater vigor in the evening for those who prefer nighttime lovemaking out of choice rather than by default. Experimenting with new times on weekends, holidays, and vacations can be invigorating. When vacations away from home are not possible, take a vacation at home. If you have the house to yourself, unplug the phone and let the outside world know you're not available. Then settle down and enjoy yourself.

Relaxation is quite conducive for putting you in the mood for romance. A warm bath or shower before sex can help, as can exchanging massages with your partner, turning the lights low, and listening to music. (Massage courses for couples are now available in many major cities as part of adult education programs.) A *small* glass of an alcoholic beverage can be a tension reliever—we recommend dry white wine or warm Japanese sake. Warm milk, while it may not be the world's sexiest drink, can be soothing as well.

What You Can Do for Your Partner

You can acquire an extensive technical knowledge about how to make love from books, tapes, lectures, and courses. (We've included some of the books on sexual technique in the Bibliography.) In our opinion, however, the *technique* of sex has been overpromoted, making lovemaking seem more like a gymnastic workout than an expression of love. Naturally, you can learn much that is valuable, but always remember that skill and technique can *never* substitute for genuine warmth and affection.

What we do want to do is direct your attention to information that is especially relevant to older people. For older women, the most common sexual problem is the inability to achieve orgasm. "Frigidity" is the word often used to describe this situation, but it is an unfortunate term because it implies coldness and sexual indifference. This does not adequately or appropriately explain what happens to many women. Women who ordinarily are able to have orgasms will have times when they are unresponsive (luckily such times are usually short-lived), and their temporary loss of response can have many causes, among them tiredness, emotional upset, boredom, vaginal infections or other physical ailments, drugs, and lack of adequate stimulation of the clitoris. Also, the loss of estrogen during menopause can affect a woman's sexual response. In addition, numbers of women never attain orgasm through intercourse but can reach it through other means, such as petting or self-stimulation. Orgasm by any of these means is enjoyable. Others never manage to reach orgasm through any method, including masturbation. Their severe or total lack of sexual response is ongoing, and can usually be traced to emotional attitudes that developed during the early years of life. For some women this condition is extremely troubling; for others mildly so; and the remainder do not consider it to be a problem at all. For those who desire to change this situation, it may be possible to do so, even at a late point in life. What can make the difference? A helpful and thoughtful partner, and/or professional counseling or sex therapy.

As to pleasing your partner, there is growing evidence that women may have a different view of sexuality from men, with women placing less importance on the act of sexual intercourse itself and more on the cuddling, physical holding, talking, and sharing that may surround a sexual relationship. While there's no indication that women are less interested than men in achieving orgasm and sexual release, many women prefer sexual activities other than, or in addition to, intercourse. Female anatomy plays an important role in women's attitudes. The majority of women receive their primary sexual satisfaction from clitoral stimulation, and that direct or indirect clitoral stimulation is the initial requirement in producing female orgasm. Because of this, sexual intercourse is often not satisfying unless it involves direct manual stimulation of the clitoris. (A number of studies indicate that substantially fewer women achieve orgasm regularly through sexual intercourse than through other methods.) Men can learn to stimulate the clitoral area, whether by hand, by mouth, or by the penis itself, and women should tell them what is pleasurable and what is not. Finally, many older women have problems of lubrication and may require longer periods of sex play before lubrication actually begins. K-Y jelly or other water-based lubricants can be used in the vagina if lubrication is insufficient.

Women can and should learn to be sensitive and helpful when men are having problems with impotence. Try a new coital position by bending your knees and placing a pillow under your hips to elevate your pelvis, in order to more easily accommodate your partner's partially erect penis. Remember that erection can be stimulated by touching the penis, so learn to massage it. Do not pull it up toward the abdomen, where it will lose blood. Instead, push down, with pressure at the base of the penis, which will put pressure on major blood vessels to hold the blood that the penis already contains.

A woman can further the strength of an erection by literally stuffing the partially erect penis into her vagina and flexing her vaginal muscles until it achieves full erection. Many women like to hold the penis in their vagina after lovemaking. If they have developed their vaginal muscles, this may be possible even if the penis begins to become limp, as happens more quickly after orgasm as men grow older. Finally, we want to stress again that a woman need not feel obligated to "give a man an orgasm" every time they make love. Leave this up to the man to decide and concentrate on mutually enjoying the physical and emotional contact, as well as your own orgasm if it occurs.

Men and women can learn to accommodate each other's needs in other ways. If one of you is obese or has a protruding abdomen, for example, you will need to experiment to find a sexual position that allows the penis to reach the vagina. One accessible position is for the man to lie on his back while the woman sits astride him.

Today older people experiment more with various sexual positions, just as do the young. There are many alternatives to the standard missionary position of the woman underneath, on her back, and the man on top. The most common ones to consider are lying side by side; the woman on top; or the man entering the woman from the rear.

As we have indicated, there are also a number of satisfying sexual alternatives to intercourse. These include mutual stimulation of each other's genitals by hand as well as stimulation of other erotic areas of the body—the mouth, neck, ears, breasts, and buttocks. Some couples use these techniques as foreplay before intercourse. Others use them as substitutes, either because intercourse is not possible or because they prefer them.

Sex gadgets are generally a waste of money except for battery-driven vibrators, which many people find stimulating, and certain prosthetic devices, which can help a man maintain a rigid penis or which can substitute completely for one. Older women should avoid douching after sex with perfumed douches or using vaginal sprays. They are unnecessary and can cause infections.

SOLO SEX

Self-stimulation, or masturbation, is a common and healthy practice that usually begins in childhood. It is natural for all children to explore their bodies, and most children stimulate themselves sexually unless they are prevented by adults from doing so. There is evidence that self-stimulation is an important preliminary to adult sexuality, enabling people to learn to recognize and satisfy their sexual feelings. The 1990 Merck Manual, a highly reputable source of medical information, reports that approximately 97 percent of males and 80 percent of females have masturbated at some point in their lives. The evidence seems clear that, although masturbation was once seen as a perversion and a cause of mental and physical disease, it is now recognized as a normal sexual activity that one can engage in throughout one's life.

Self-stimulation provides a sexual outlet for people—unmarried, widowed, or divorced—who do not have partners, as well as for husbands or wives whose partners are ill or away. Some people practice self-stimulation in addition to sexual intercourse, particularly if they prefer sex more frequently than their partner does or enjoy the variety masturbation affords. And as described earlier, many women experience more intense and more frequent orgasms through self-masturbation or mutual masturbation with their partners than during intercourse. Masturbation can continue until very late in life and has been reported by some men in their nineties. A 1983 Consumers Union survey found that 66 percent of men and 47 percent of women in their fifties masturbate with some regularity; over the age of seventy, 43 percent of men and 33 percent of women still masturbate. In fact, some people begin to masturbate for the first time after they grow older, particularly if they have no partner or become too physically incapacitated for intercourse.

Total abstinence from sexual activity over a period of time can be tension-producing and may result in potency problems in men and loss of lubrication as well as vaginal shape in women. So it can be beneficial to free yourself from the notion that self-stimulation is unhealthy, immoral, or immature. A source of pleasure to be learned and enjoyed for its own sake, masturbation also resolves sexual tensions, keeps sexual desire alive, is good physical exercise, and helps to preserve sexual functioning in both men and women who have no other outlets. Vibrators can be useful aids in masturbation. Many people engage in sexual fantasies, which add to the pleasure of self-stimulation.

COMMUNICATING WITH YOUR PARTNER ABOUT SEX

It's often extremely helpful to talk with your partner about your sexual feelings. Many couples assume at first that they don't have to talk, since sex "comes naturally," but this is simply not accurate. Because people are all different, with unique likes and dislikes, it is naive to assume that our partners can read our minds or know intuitively how to please us. Furthermore, it is often said that sex begins in the brain, by the stimulation of the imagination and by memory of previous sexual experience. Our mind may well be our most sensitive and reliable organ of sensuality, so you should exercise it.

Begin by discussing your feelings about talking

about sex. It may seem embarrassing or awkward at first, but it's usually worth it to continue. Then tell your partner what gives you pleasure and have him or her do likewise. Finally, try in every way possible to do what is pleasurable for each other. You may be surprised at what you don't know about your partner and what you may have been reluctant to admit about yourself. You can also reminisce, talking about your first memories of sex, your early sexual attitudes and those of your family, and perhaps your feelings about what it means to be a man or a woman. Compare notes on what you would most like to change about yourself and your partner sexually. However, do be thoughtful and kind about the way you express any dissatisfactions you may feel.

Some couples go so far as to share their sexual fantasies with each other. Such fantasies, which are part of most people's sex lives, involve any visual and sexually stimulating images one conjures up. Some people are excited by imagining forbidden or unavailable sex partners, settings, or practices. Others bring to mind sexual experiences from the past that have been especially exciting. Some couples even make up fantasies for each other. The use of sexual videotapes at home may enhance fantasy and sexual stimulation.

The value of fantasy is that it adds a new dimension to one's sex life. People who may be otherwise fond of their partners but not easily aroused by them as the years go by report that fantasies, including fantasies of their partners and themselves when they were younger ("fantasy reruns"), can often get things started and help in reaching orgasms. Use fantasy to override a physical disability or distract yourself from anxiety or other preoccupations. Mental imaging can be especially useful for those whose vision is impaired. Since poor vision can interfere with the vital transfer of visual stimuli into sexual arousal, fantasy may provide the means for recapturing that stimuli.

So far we have few useful studies about fantasy in mid and later life. It would be interesting, for example, to know whether people usually fantasize themselves and others as younger than their actual ages.

Peruse books on sexuality and emotional relationships to learn more about yourself and each other. It is useful and stimulating to take a fresh look from time to time at what you know about sexuality and at the current attitudes of society toward sex. We have recommended a number of books in the Bibliography. (There are many more, but most of them assume a young and middle-aged readership.) There are now films and tapes specifically addressed to medical and other aspects of sexuality in the mid and later years that are available to both health-care professionals and the public. Seek these out as well.

CHAPTER 9

❧❧

DATING, REMARRIAGE, AND YOUR CHILDREN

Many conflicts develop between parents and their adult children when a widowed or divorced parent attempts to build a new life through dating and, possibly, remarriage. To wit: "My daughter doesn't like my fiancée and thinks she is only interested in my money." "My son Jim feels I'd be a fool to marry Harry, since Harry has always been a ladies' man." "My children think I'm crazy to want a man. I wouldn't dare tell them what I did on my cruise to Jamaica."

Not all children create such problems. Many are pleased and, indeed, relieved at the thought of their parents leading full and satisfying lives. Others have realistic worries about the practical implications of these new life-styles; they may welcome the remarriage of a

246

father to a somewhat younger woman, because she will be able to nurse him as he grows older, but may feel threatened if their mother marries an older man, because it will be a burden on her, and potentially on them if he should fall ill.

For still other children the reactions are entirely emotional. The thought of a parent becoming involved with a new partner can provoke such strong emotions as anxiety, jealousy, hurt, fear, anger, or grief. In response they may be strongly inclined to offer unasked-for advice and even to "take over" if they feel a parent is making a mistake. Resorting to coercion, threats, and angry withdrawal are not at all uncommon.

As to why adult children react so negatively, there are numerous reasons. Those who never became fully independent psychologically use their parents to fulfill emotional needs that should be met by their partners and friends. You can assume this is the case if your child acts possessive or personally aggrieved, not unlike a wounded lover, when you become involved in a relationship. It is possible that you yourself (perhaps unconsciously) have encouraged an inappropriately close relationship with this child, or that other circumstances have kept the child from emancipating him- or herself. Age does not factor into these situations. Your fifty-year-old child can be dependent in this way even though he or she is married and has children. Under these circumstances, the best approach is to let your children know, kindly but definitely, that you intend to lead your own life, and to encourage them to do likewise.

Sometimes parents find that their children cling to the parental image of you as Mom or Dad and do not recognize (or want to recognize) that you need love and sex just as they do. Probably you have encouraged this attitude yourself by playing only the parent role whenever you were around them. A good antidote is to tell them more about your social interests and to bring your friends and dates home to meet them. You can still retain your privacy, but they should become aware that you are entitled to emotional and personal commitments. Though they may never feel entirely at ease about your right to a sexually satisfying life, they can often be helped to come to terms with its reality.

Children will sometimes try to preserve the memory of their deceased parent (or of your former relationship with a divorced spouse) by the process of *enshrinement,* discussed earlier in terms of widowhood. They maintain a fierce reverence for the past and want to see nothing changed, so any new relationships you enter into they consider an affront to their other parent. They may then accuse you of being selfish, insensitive, or disloyal; and if they succeed in making you feel guilty, you may be compelled to sever your new relationship. *This is a mistake.* Your children need to work through their own anger and grief at the death (or divorce) that ended your marriage. They are often bound to the past by a mixture of positive and negative feelings, and it is this ambivalence that must be resolved. Talk to them about their feelings, listen to their reactions, and try honestly to answer questions and clarify confusion. Also, let them know how you have handled your own feelings about their other parent.

Another problem can develop if your children have grievances or hold grudges against you, which they demonstrate by refusing to condone your right to build a new life for yourself. Some of these grievances may be lifelong, others recent; some may be misconceptions and misunderstandings of your actions toward them (particularly during their childhood), and others may be legitimate. Adult children easily become critical of their parents if their parents were always critical of them. Others remember being harshly punished or humiliated for innocent sexual experiences in childhood and have grown up thinking sex is wrong or dirty—and this might now include the sex lives of their parents. If you can begin listening openly to their grievances—even though it may be difficult—there is a chance that you and your children can develop a new understanding and respect for each other. Be ready to admit where you may have failed, but don't take the blame for everything. Your children and your former partner played their roles too. The point is not to pin down a culprit, find a "bad guy," or allay grievances by making yourself a martyr, but to clarify what happened, why it happened, and whether anything can now be done to build a better relationship.

Frank talk itself sometimes heals old wounds. And when it doesn't, *you* decide what choice you are going to make.

Next we must look at a problem that can terrorize a parent—the spoiled child. This is the child who grows up believing himself or herself to be inordinately important and never stops believing it. Every spoiled child has one and usually two parents who were easily intimidated, overindulgent, or lax with discipline. A favorite tactic of such a child is to threaten to withdraw love if the parent does not cater to his or her wishes. This tactic is all the more devastating when the child grows to middle age and attains greater power as the parent becomes older and loses status and authority. The sooner you get a hold on this situation, the better. *Do not let your son or daughter dictate to you.* It isn't good for you, and it certainly isn't good for your child. It may be frightening to think of losing this love, but remember that children rarely "divorce" their parents (if they do so, it's usually for a limited period of time, to try to get their own way), particularly if they know that basically you care about them.

Spoiled children have an intuitive understanding of power; they learned to use it expertly at a very early age. Use power in your turn to let them know the score. First of all, *keep your grip on your own money and property.* Then start making a few of your own decisions, particularly about your personal life. Get outside authority figures to help you if you need them in the initial battles that are bound to come. Your lawyer, your cleric, or a respected friend or family member may be able to support you when you waver, or speak for you if at first you can't. Be heartened by the knowledge that spoiled children usually develop respect for people who refuse to be manipulated.

Finally, we come to a most painful problem: the child who has one eye on your will. He or she is found particularly in those families where there will be a sizable estate after a parent's death. This child is forever worrying about his or her share of your estate and casts a cold eye on anyone you may be dating or thinking of marrying. Such a child will often plant suspicions in your mind that any close friend or prospective mate is after whatever money you have. Unfortunately, this happened to an attractive and vigorous widow we knew named Margaret. She had known Nathan only a short time and was surprised at how happy she felt when she realized that he was in the same room, or when his name was mentioned. She hadn't felt that way since her husband's courtship during their youth. Nathan and Margaret began to date and, eventually, to talk of marriage. However, to Nathan's astonishment, as soon as the talk turned to marriage, his children became extremely negative toward Margaret. They told their father that they were sure that she was a gold digger. He was horrified, but he had always trusted his children's opinions and so decided to hold off on marriage for a while. In turn, Margaret was justifiably hurt, and Nathan's decision changed their relationship. She felt wrongfully accused. Nevertheless, Nathan could not proceed wholeheartedly without his children's acceptance. The impasse finally gave way to alienation, and Nathan and Margaret sadly went their separate ways.

Don't let this happen to you. While older people can be and have been exploited, if your mind is sound, you should rely on your own judgment and perhaps that of trusted friends or advisers—*not* on a child with a reputation for an obsessive focus on money or an inclination to avarice. (If you begin to have any questions about your own judgment, you can seek legal advice to set up a conservatorship. This will protect you, your funds, and your estate.)

What makes a child obsessive about his or her inheritance? Many things: parental overindulgence, feelings of being unloved, a long-standing family overemphasis on money, a lack of funds, or a lack of training in the pleasure there is in generosity and sharing with others. Simple selfishness and greed also exist. This is a difficult problem to rectify unless your child is motivated to discover the basis of his or her attitudes toward material possessions. Try to understand any part you may have played in shaping these attitudes and see what changes you can make in them. But also protect yourself financially and emotionally from capitulating to your child's demands. *Your estate is your own to disperse as you see fit.* If your son or daughter puts the pressure on, it may help to keep the provisions of your will secret. If your child is capable of maintaining some rationality in this area, however, it may be helpful to say exactly what you intend to do so that he or she can learn to live with it. The important thing is to be decisive and remain unintimidated by veiled or open threats, pressures, and pleadings focused upon your property.

In general, your children's emotional reactions toward your personal life are likely to run deep. They require your special attention if you are to avoid unnecessary alienation and hostility. Family councils and heart-to-heart talks can help enormously. But if all else fails, look for professional advice and try to get your children to join you. If they refuse, seek help by yourself, but make it clear to your children (and to yourself) that you are working toward their eventual acceptance of your new life.

Prenuptial Legal Planning

For those of you who have decided on a marriage, prenuptial legal planning is advisable and often essential. We will focus on only one important form of such planning, the prenuptial agreement or contract, also called a premarital or antenuptial agreement. (Do not confuse it with modern marriage contracts, which stipulate marital duties and are not legally binding.) Prenuptial agreements deal only with money and other property. You may also want to consider alternative forms (trusts, for example), but these are beyond the scope of this book. Whatever kind of prenuptial planning you elect will require consultation with a lawyer.

Many parents want to leave at least part of their estate directly to their children and become concerned about the effects of remarriage on this intention. If you are planning to remarry and want to make special financial arrangements for the benefit of your children or any other persons, you and your spouse-to-be can work out a prenuptial agreement. In most states these agreements are a time-honored method for allaying the fears of children and planning one's estate wisely and in their best interests. Such agreements also protect you by keeping your resources intact and unavailable to anyone but those whom you have designated. Wealthy people of all ages have traditionally used prenuptial agreements to protect their estates. Now, with people living longer, with more late-life marriages, and with more extensive estates to dispose of, prenuptial agreements are increasingly common. The agreement customarily describes what will *not* be available to the prospective spouse.

To be legally enforceable, such an agreement must be in writing, by reason of the Statute of Frauds in force in all states. The Uniform Premarital Agreement Act, approved by the American Bar Association in February

1984, can be used as a model for a premarital agreement. Since it's a basic agreement acceptable in all states, it is likely to stand up in court. For copies of the agreement, ask your lawyer or contact your local chapter of the American Bar Association.

How does a prenuptial agreement work? Let's take as an example a couple who plan to marry, each of whom has been widowed and has children. The prenuptial agreement enables them to plan their respective estates in the way that best suits them. The advantage to the children lies in the fact that their parent's new spouse will receive an amount less than ordinary under the Statute of Descent and Distributions and the children will receive more. An added advantage is that under such an agreement the children will receive somewhat more than if the parent had died intestate (without a will).

A prenuptial agreement *is* different from a will. It is a waiver to the right of the spouse to a certain minimum claim to your property at death. A will can be changed at any time without the spouse's knowledge or consent; a prenuptial agreement can be amended *only* with the consent of both parties. It is binding as soon as the marriage takes place; a will goes into effect only at the time of death. A will can, of course, be changed to give a spouse more and the children less than what the prenuptial agreement stated. But unless the will stipulates this, the spouse cannot lay claim to any more than what the prenuptial agreement provides for.

Prenuptial agreements are useful even though estates may be small. Take, as an example, a widower of moderate assets with children by his first wife, who had assisted him in earning the money he has accumulated and whose children contributed actively as well. Now that he wants to remarry, there is some resentment on the part of the children that the new bride will be automatically entitled to one-third (or whatever proportion is operative in a particular state) of their father's entire estate in the event of his death. If he chooses to do so, the father can decide on a prenuptial agreement that provides something less than one-third of the estate for the new wife, with the rest going to children or grandchildren. The financial gain to the children may be small, but emotionally it may mean a great deal.

There are situations where prenuptial agreements have been challenged, and the courts have in some cases upheld those challenges if fraud was involved or certain formalities had not been observed. The law says that the contracting parties must be in a confidential (or fiduciary) relationship to each other, meaning that there *must* be a good-faith disclosure of assets. For example, suppose a man who has several hundred thousand dollars tells his bride-to-be he has only twenty thousand dollars; she agrees on the basis of his statement to take the sum of five thousand dollars in the event of his death. His failure to reveal the truth makes the agreement subject to challenge on the basis of fraud.

Another problem arises from separation or divorce. Prenuptial agreements provide for the eventuality of death, and these agreements are expressly recognized in about one-fourth of the states by statute and in most of the other states by judicial decision. When the agreement deals not only with the division of property in the event of death, but with the possibility of divorce as well, you may encounter problems. For example, many states hold that agreements entered into before marriage to provide for divorce payments (in the event of separation) are invalid. However, a Washington, D.C. District Court of Appeals decision *(Burtoff* v. *Burtoff)* upheld this broadening of a prenuptial agreement as it related to alimony and property settlements. Nonetheless, many agreements have been thrown out or modified by the courts after one of the parties has accused the other of coercion. To minimize such challenges, make certain that you draw up an agreement well in advance of the wedding, in order to avoid charges of duress. And *never* force such an agreement upon your partner. It must be a mutual understanding that both wish to participate.

So how much should you tell your children about your prenuptial agreement, or the making or changing of your will? Some parents inform each child fully or have their lawyer do so. Others give a general picture but not the specifics. Still others keep everything totally secret. What you do depends on your own judgment.

Children may be relieved to have at least a general idea of your intentions. But if privacy about your own financial affairs is important to you, you have every right to keep the arrangements to yourself.

CHAPTER 10

❧ ～ ❧

WHERE TO GO
FOR HELP

We have discussed throughout this book what older people can do for themselves to understand and remedy sexual, personal, and social problems. But when such problems persist, it's a good idea to seek outside professional help.

A thorough evaluation is crucial to determining exactly where the problem lies. And the first step in any evaluation of sexual problems in your age group should *always* be a medical examination. Physical problems can cause serious sexual difficulties by themselves, or they can team up with emotional or social problems to create quite a baffling group of sexual symptoms. Unraveling the medical aspects of sexual problems may be simple, or it may be terribly complicated; in either case, it should not be neglected.

FINDING MEDICAL HELP

How do you find a doctor who is knowledgeable about sex? More specifically, how do you find one who is interested in older people and who understands the special problems of sex in later life? Frankly, it may be very difficult. Many doctors—especially those graduating from medical school before 1961—have not had sex education as part of their medical school training. While this has slowly changed, you will still find that many doctors are surprisingly unenlightened and embarrassed to talk about sexual activity throughout the course of one's life. Many draw primarily upon their own personal sexual philosophy and experience. (This is especially true about sex in the later years.) They may also personally share the culture's negative attitude toward old age. It is not uncommon for women past fifty who see only an internist or a family practitioner (rather than a gynecologist) to find that their doctor begins to "forget" to do a thorough gynecological exam during a routine physical examination.

Adding to the difficulty of a search for a sympathetic and knowledgeable doctor is the fact that most doctors have not had systematic training in the general medical problems of older people. This also is slowly changing and some medical school programs have begun to include geriatrics—the prevention, cure, and treatment of the problems of older people—in their curricula, but lack of knowledge and interest remains widespread among practicing physicians. Two national organizations, the American Geriatrics Society (770 Lexington Avenue, Suite 400, New York, NY 10021) and the Gerontological Society of America's Clinical Medicine Section (1411 K Street, N.W., Suite 300, Washington, DC 20005) may be able to help you locate doctors in your area who are knowledgeable in geriatrics. You can also write the Office of Information of the National Institute on Aging (National Institutes of Health, Bethesda, MD 20205) or the National Institute of Mental Health (National Institutes of Health, Rockville, MD 20857) for a list of doctors or clinics specializing in geriatrics and gerontology arranged by geographical area. Now doctors, after taking an exam, can obtain a Certificate of Competence in geriatrics, within the specialties of internal medicine, family practice, and psychiatry. Ask your doctor if he or she is so certified.

Still, it is wise to remember, that there is an extremely small percentage of doctors active in this field. It is also true that membership in these organizations does not guarantee competence in the field of aging, and individual doctors who are not specialists in the field may be equally sensitive and knowledgeable in working with older people. An able and understanding general practitioner or internist who takes care of patients of all ages can serve you very well indeed. If you are lucky, your own doctor may be such a person. Some people, of course, feel more comfortable talking about sexual problems with a new doctor who is a total stranger, and if this is the case with you, by all means do so. The main point is to go to a doctor with whom you feel as relaxed as possible and whom you trust to be both medically competent and generally receptive toward older people.

What else can you do? You owe it to yourself to learn how to give proper information and ask the right questions, and thus encourage your doctor to take your sexual problems seriously. It may be embarrassing to talk about what is on your mind, but don't let that stop you. Your experiences and problems are shared by many older people. Tell the doctor *exactly* what you are worried about. Include any detail that you think might be helpful in evaluating the symptoms. Older women may feel reluctant to describe sexual problems in general, or problems in the vaginal area in particular, especially to a male doctor. Older men may not want to admit problems with potency. But this is false modesty and false pride. Candid talk will go a long way toward making it easier to diagnose and treat your problem.

There are a number of things you should look for as you work with doctors:

• Beware of any doctor who quickly dismisses your sexual concerns with such comments as "What do you expect at your age?" "Go home and take a cold shower," "Stop worrying," or "Nothing can be done." Persist in your desire for help; if the doctor continues to be unresponsive, find a new doctor.

• Expect the doctor to take a good medical history, which includes a review of the body's systems and functions as well as a history of present and past illnesses. Specifically, the doctor should ask you about any changes you have observed in your genital organs, including in men any bowing of the penis and in women stress incontinence.

• Be aware that not only do diseases affect sexuality but the proper control of disease may, in many instances, restore good sexual functioning.

• Expect the doctor to take a thorough sexual and marital history as well as a medical history. Questions are likely to cover the ways you and your partner feel about sex, its frequency and pleasure, and any disagreements you may have. The doctor will also explore the impact of attitudes toward sex you may have developed in childhood. You will find it valuable to share with your doctor the history of sexual experiences you may have had with people at other times. Male patients should be asked if they have problems with urination and with achieving and holding erections. They should be questioned as to whether they ever have erections as they wake up in the morning. Females should be questioned carefully as to whether they are having any pain during intercourse or any unusual soreness or bleeding.

• The doctor should ask what drugs you are taking, both prescription and over-the-counter, and be able to explain the sexual side effects of each drug. It is sometimes possible to switch to equally effective drugs with fewer sexual side effects.

• If you have already had surgery on any sex organs, the doctor should be able to tell you if this is in any way affecting your sexuality. If surgery is planned, learn in advance about any possible sexual consequences. Do not be embarrassed to ask specific questions about anything that is troubling you.

• Discuss with your doctor a program of preventive health care. This should include attention to smoking, drinking, nutrition, exercise, rest, stress, and emotional problems.

• Using these questions and the doctor's reactions to you as a guide, and relying as well on your own common sense, if you feel your doctor's examination has been insufficient, talk to him or her openly about your misgivings. As a patient, you are entitled to satisfaction.

• Review insurance payment procedures with your doctor. Many types of diagnostic and treatment procedures are now reimbursable under insurance programs, including Medicare.

• Finally, your doctor should ask if you have any questions.

After the medical examination it should be fairly clear whether physical problems are the sole or, more likely, the partial cause of symptoms of sexual dysfunction and whether medical treatment is indicated. The point of the medical examination is to find out whether bodily changes are involved significantly or not at all; if they are not, or they have only a minor significance, the search for the causes of sexual problems must move to emotional or psychological areas.

FINDING PSYCHOLOGICAL HELP

Most sexual problems have emotional components, even when the original cause is physical, and some are entirely emotional in origin. Much of what we have said about the competence and inclinations of medical doctors with regard to older people also holds true for psychotherapists and counselors. They tend to be unaware of and at times uninterested in the emotional problems of later life. They have usually had some training in sex education but rarely in the specialized area of sex after sixty. To find a therapist who can be of help to you will probably require major determination.

The following is a classic humorous story that exposes some of the false assumptions about the elderly and their sexuality: A couple well into their eighties visited a sex therapist asking for a consultation. The therapist suggested that they might be at the wrong place and explained that his job was to help people with sexual problems. "But that's why we're here," the husband emphasized. The therapist proceeded to ask skeptically, "When was the first time you noticed this sexual problem?" "Why, last night," the wife replied matter-of-factly, "and then again this morning."

That said, there are several types of therapy to choose from. *Individual psychotherapy* means talking with a therapist one-to-one on a regular basis. *Marital counseling* involves both you and your partner. A broader term is *couples therapy*, which encompasses unmarried couples as well. *Family counseling* means the inclusion of other members of your family. *Psychoanalysis* is an intensive form of individual psychotherapy, requiring several sessions a week. *Group psychotherapy* usually consists of a group of five to ten patients whose problems are discussed by the group under the guidance of one or two therapists. *Sex therapy* is a relatively new specialty, which concentrates on the actual sexual problem itself, teaching couples how to make love more effectively.

The background and training of therapists vary greatly. Psychotherapists can be *psychiatrists* (M.D.s who specialize in psychiatry), *psychologists* (with master's or doctoral degrees in psychology), or *social workers* (with master's or doctoral degrees in social work). (The term "social worker" can be confusing, since people may define themselves as social workers because of the kind of work they do rather than because of their training. Ask if the social worker has, at minimum, a master's degree in social work.) *Psychoanalysts* have had advanced training in the psychoanalytic method. All these fields require a program of formal education and a supervised training period in psychotherapy or casework. All states require doctors to be licensed, and this is beginning to be true for practicing psychologists and social workers as well. Social workers who are certified (you will see the letters A.C.S.W.—for Academy of Certified Social Workers—after their names) by the National Association of Social Workers have had a period of professional training and examination beyond the master's degree. A number of states also have a special certification for advanced clinical social workers.

In addition to psychotherapists, there are numerous other kinds of counselors. *Marriage counselors* work with marriage and sex problems. This is a still unregulated field and practitioners range from competent and well-trained professionals to quacks and charlatans. Be careful to investigate the credentials (professional training and experience) of anyone you are considering as a counselor. *Pastoral counseling* has grown out of the counseling role of the clergy, with individual clerics counseling, supervising, and training others to counsel. The quality of this counseling depends on the training and skills of each individual; there are no standard requirements for such training in theological schools.

Well-trained *sex therapists* are usually much more able than other health professionals to evaluate and help resolve specific sexual problems. A general rule is that if you are seeing your family doctor, cleric, etc., regarding sexual problems, a resolution to your problems should begin to occur in six to eight sessions. If it doesn't you should seek referral to a specialist in sex therapy. *All About Sex Therapy* by Peter R. Kilmann, M.D., and Katherine H. Mills, M.D. (Plenum Press, 1983) will help answer your questions about how sex therapy works.

Sex therapists have proliferated in recent years. Following Masters and Johnson's important clinical work in the treatment of sexual dysfunction, thousands of practitioners now offer such therapy. But many are untrained or poorly trained, and some are outright frauds. Because this is a new field, without an organized and uniform structure of qualifications, requirements, examinations, clinical experience, or peer review (licensing laws vary from state to state)—and because sexual problems are so susceptible to exploitation by skillful, smooth-talking incompetents—the choice of a sex counselor requires very careful consideration.

How do you find competent psychotherapists, counselors, and sex therapists? Some sources to check are university medical schools and clinical teaching hospitals (many have sex therapy clinics); local medical or psychiatric societies; university schools of social work; community mental health centers; senior centers; local chapters of the National Association of Social Workers, Inc. (write to 750 First Street, N.E., Washington, DC 20002 for a listing of local chapters); the American Psychological Association (write to 1200 17th Street, N.W., Washington, DC 20036 for a list of psychological associations in your state); the National Mental Health Association (write to 1021 Prince Street, Alexandria, VA 22314 for a list of local chapters); Family Service America (to find its member Family Service agencies write to 11700 West Lake Park Drive, Milwaukee, WI 53224); and your family doctor or cleric.

When talking to these suggested sources, be specific and ask for a therapist who will be interested in working with an older person in sex counseling. Ask for at least two names so you will be able to make a choice. Friends and acquaintances may be able to refer you to professionals who have been helpful to them, as long as you recognize that individual preferences vary considerably.

The National Institute of Mental Health's Center on Aging (9000 Rockville Pike, Bethesda, MD 20892) and the Gerontological Society's Social Research, Planning and Practice Section (1411 K Street, N.W., Suite

300, Washington, DC 20005) can be contacted for information. The American Association for Marriage and Family Therapy (1100 17th Street, N.W., 10th floor, Washington, DC 20036) is pressing for regulation of persons who call themselves marriage counselors and should be able to refer you to someone in your locale (including Canada). The American Association of Sex Educators, Counselors, and Therapists (435 North Michigan Avenue, Suite 1717, Chicago, IL 60611) certifies sex counselor–therapists and has a national roster from which names can be obtained. You may want to write the Masters and Johnson Institute (24 South Kingshighway, St. Louis, MO 63108) for referral to competent sex counselors near you who have been trained by them. The Sex Information and Education Council of the United States (SIECUS) (32 Washington Place, Room 52, New York University, New York, NY 10003) is an additional source of information and referral.

The cost of therapy varies from free clinics and free counseling, to sliding fees based on income, up to $150 or more for a fifty-minute session (in 1992). Group therapy is less costly than individual therapy. Some health insurance plans partially cover costs of psychotherapy. Many do not. Medicare now pays 50 percent of the allowable charge for psychotherapy, whether performed by physicians, psychologists, or social workers. Few insurance programs cover sex therapy per se. However, the Diagnostic and Statistical Manual of Mental

Disorders (DSM-III-R) categorizes sexual dysfunctions under the following: Sexual Desire Disorders; Sexual Arousal Disorders; Orgasm Disorders; and Sexual Pain Disorders. Some insurance companies will reimburse if a specific DSM-III-R diagnosis is used. So ask your therapist if such a diagnosis may be relevant for you and you may be reimbursed for at least part of your costs.

The amount of time required for evaluating and, if possible, resolving a particular sexual problem varies. Sometimes a single session can be enough. More often a series of weekly sessions is recommended, lasting from several months to more than a year or, in the case of psychoanalysis, a number of years.

WHAT HAPPENS IN PSYCHOTHERAPY?

You can't literally change the past, obviously, but you can gain perspective about it, change the way you feel about it, and break old habits and acquire new ways of coping effectively. Through talking about and exploring your past patterns, you come to understand the sources of sexual problems, lose certain inhibitions, and learn new avenues of sexual expression. Therapeutic counseling does not simply dwell on the past, however. You will also be discussing the here and now, your present relationships. Your therapist will ask questions, make comments (some may startle you), and propose suggestions.

Working out conflicts and going in new directions, therefore, come about through joint work by you *and* your therapist on the past and the present. Together you work on your private life.

The process itself may remind you of both parenting and teaching. You retain your basic personality, but hopefully you rid yourself of unwelcome symptoms, gain insight and enhanced well-being, and increase your effectiveness in everyday living. Altogether you are likely to feel better about yourself.

How should you act when you go to the therapist? Once again, be frank. Tell him or her whatever is troubling you. There are certain basic things you can require or expect:

• Your therapist needs to be well informed both about the problems of older people and about sexual problems. Don't be afraid to question therapists about their background, training, and general interest in these areas. Evaluate their answers (or failures to answer) in terms of what you now know—from this book and from your own experiences—to be important to you.

• The therapist should ask for your sexual, marital, and personal history, and probably will want a medical report from your doctor.

• You should feel a sense of rapport and comfort with the therapist by the time you have had several sessions. If not, discuss your feelings frankly. If matters do not improve, you may need to consider a different therapist, since rapport and trust are crucial to effectively working out sexual and emotional problems. However, do not consider the need to change therapists to be the result of a flaw in yourself. Each individual's requirements in a relationship as close as that of therapist and patient will be different, and intangible but crucial factors like empathy, perception, manner, and attitude are involved in making the right choice. A personality and approach that are right for one person may be all wrong for another. As long as you are candid in your encounters with the therapist, trust in your own perceptions about whether he or she is a good choice for you.

As for your part in the therapy, you must learn to:

• Set aside shyness and embarrassment.
• Open your mind and feelings to new ideas and insights.
• Be willing to actively try new directions in your relationships with others.
• Realize that while many things can improve, some things cannot. Once you have decided—with the aid of your therapist—which is which, you can begin to work on those areas where improvement can realistically occur.

WHAT HAPPENS IN SEX THERAPY?

Sex therapy is a unique, usually short-term form of therapy that has evolved over the past thirty years under the leadership of Dr. William Masters and Virginia Johnson of St. Louis. This method is quite effective in rapidly treating problems like premature ejaculation, vaginal spasm, failure to achieve orgasm, and some forms of impotence. It is much more difficult, but not always impossible, to treat low or absent sexual desire or lack of pleasure in sex. (Low sexual desire usually requires longer-term and more intensive psychotherapy.) "Desire discrepancy," which occurs when one partner wishes to have sex more (or less) frequently than the other, is another common problem that can often be resolved in this kind of therapy.

The original Masters and Johnson sex therapy techniques required a male and female therapist for each couple, a two-week stay in a hotel near the treatment center (so the couple was isolated and could concentrate on therapy), and daily therapy sessions. Patients were provided with two years of follow-up assistance from therapists available twenty-four hours a day (usually by telephone), for no extra charge. Most sex therapists now have modified this so that couples can remain in their own communities and homes and have therapy once or twice a week for about fourteen sessions. Educational counseling about sex, improving communication between a couple, and carrying out "pleasuring exercises" are all part of treatment.

Therapists may use movies and slides in their teaching, as well as group therapy. Couples with marital problems that go beyond their sexual difficulties are encouraged to obtain marital counseling and/or individual psychotherapy. Also, you should know that individuals who are not part of a couple are also accepted for sex therapy.

In summary, we'd like to make very clear that even sexual problems that have existed for many years have the possibility of resolution. This is true whether your sexual problems are new or long-term. As long as they are troubling to you, you owe it to yourself to see what can be done to resolve them. In many cases you will be happy with the results.

CHAPTER 11

❧❧

THE SECOND
LANGUAGE OF SEX

Can sex really remain interesting and exciting after forty, fifty, or sixty years of adulthood? Yes. Older people themselves have testified that it can. Affection, warmth, and sensuality do not have to deteriorate with age; they may, in fact, increase.

Sex in later life is sex for its own sake: pleasure, release, communication, shared intimacy. Except for older men involved with younger women, it is no longer associated with childbearing and the creation of families. This freedom can be both exhilarating and insightful, especially for those who have literally never had the time until now to think about and get to know themselves and each other.

Love and sex can mean many different things to older people:

• *The opportunity for expression of passion, affection, admiration, loyalty, and other positive emotions.* This can occur in long-term relationships that have steadily grown and developed over the years, in relationships that actually improve in later years, and in new relationships such as second or third marriages.

• *An affirmation of one's body and its functioning.* An active sex life demonstrates to older people that their bodies are still capable of working well and providing pleasure. For many people, satisfactory sexual functioning is an extremely important part of their lives and helps to maintain high morale and enthusiasm.

• *A strong sense of self.* Sexuality is one of the ways people get a sense of their identity—who they are and what their impact is on others. Positive reactions from others preserve and enhance our self-esteem. Feeling "feminine" or "masculine," whatever meaning these terms have for each individual, is connected with feeling valued as a person. Negative reactions depress and discourage older people and may tempt them to write off their sexuality forever.

• *A means of self-assertion.* The patterns of self-assertion available when people are young change as they grow older. Their children are grown-up and gone; their jobs are usually behind them; personal and social relationships now become far more important as outlets for expressing personality. Sex can be a valuable means of positive self-assertion. One man told us, "I feel like a million dollars when I make love even though we are scrimping along on Social Security. My wife has always made me feel like a great success in bed and I believe I do the same for her. We've been able to stand a lot of stress in life because of our closeness this way."

• *Protection from anxiety.* The intimacy and the closeness of sexual union bring security and significance to people's lives, particularly when the outside world threatens them with hazards and losses. An older couple we know described the warmth of their sexual life as "a port in the storm," a place to escape from worry and trouble. A very much older woman, concerned with her eventual death, called sex "the ultimate closeness against the night." Sex serves as an important means of feeling in charge when other elements of one's life feel out of control.

• *Defiance of the stereotypes of aging.* Familiar though they are with the derogatory attitudes of society toward late-life sex, older people who are sexually active defy the neutered status expected of them. We have heard them say, "We're not finished yet," "I'm not ready to kick the bucket," "You can't keep a good man [woman] down," or "There may be snow on the roof but there's still fire in the furnace." And it's true.

• *The pleasure of being touched or caressed.* Older widows, widowers, and divorced people describe how much they miss the simple pleasure and warmth of physical closeness, of being touched, held, and caressed by someone they care for. Holding and hugging friends, children, and pets offer some compensation but do not replace the special intimacy and feeling of being cared about that can exist in a good relationship or sexual union.

• *A sense of romance.* The courting aspects of sexuality may be highly significant—flowers, soft lights, music, a sense of romantic pursuit, elegance, sentiment, and courtliness—and give pleasure in themselves. Romance may continue even when sexual intercourse, for various reasons, ceases. John and Rachel, a couple in their eighties, described their evenings together to us. They typically bathe and dress for dinner, she in a long dress, he in a suit and tie. They dine with candlelight and music, listen to music during the evening, hold hands, and enjoy each other's companionship. At bedtime they fall asleep in each other's arms. Often they awaken in the middle of the night and have long, intimate conversations, sleeping late the next morning. John said of his wife, "I fall in love with her every day. My feelings grow stronger when I realize we have only a certain amount of time left."

• *An affirmation of life.* Sex expresses joy and continued affirmation of life. The quality of one's most intimate relationships is an important measure of whether life has been worthwhile. Many otherwise successful people may count their lives a failure if they have been unable to achieve significant closeness to other people, and have never felt fully desired or accepted. Conversely, people with modest accomplishments may feel highly satisfied about themselves if they have been affirmed through intimate relationships. Sexual intimacy is only one way of achieving intimacy, of course, but it is an especially profound affirmation of the worth-whileness of life.

• *A continuing search for sensual growth and experience.* Some older people continue to search throughout their lives for ways to create new excitement and experiences. Some who are dissatisfied with their present lives look for ways to improve them. Others seek marriage counseling, pursue divorce, remarriage, or new relationships in the hope of finding what they are searching for. But many can find this growth and excitement within their present relationship if they learn some of the skills that make it possible. Love and sex are twin arts: both require effort and knowledge. Only in fairy tales do people live happily ever after without working at it. It takes a continuous and active effort to master the processes that eradicate emotional distances between two people and to continue to grow and learn.

When people are young and first getting used to sexuality, their sex tends to be urgent and explosive. It's involved largely with physical pleasure and in many cases the conception of children. This is the *first language of sex*. It is biological and instinctive, wonderfully exciting and energizing. The process of discovering one's ability to be sexually desirable and sexually effective often becomes a way of asserting independence, strength, prowess, and power. The first language of sex has been much discussed and written about because it is easy to study and measure; one can tabulate physical response, frequency of contacts, forms of outlet, sexual positions, and physical skills in lovemaking. But sex is not just a matter of athletics and "production." Some people recognize this early on and simultaneously develop a *second language of sex*, which is emotional and communicative as well as physical. Others continue largely in the first language —sometimes all their lives, sometimes only until they begin to see its limitations and desire something more.

The second language is largely learned rather than instinctive and is often vastly underdeveloped, since it depends upon the ability to recognize and share feelings in words, actions, and unspoken perceptions, and to achieve mutual tenderness and thoughtfulness with another person. In its richest form, the second language becomes highly creative and imaginative, with bountiful possibilities for new emotional experiences. Yet it is a slow-developing art, acquired deliberately and painstakingly through years of experience in giving and receiving.

In the natural flow of events in the life cycle, you will eventually find yourself reevaluating many areas of your life, including your sexuality. Middle age is the period when people typically begin to take stock of their lives and reassess their work, their personal relationships, their social and spiritual commitments. Retirement is another time when such reevaluations take place. Both periods can be chaotic, generating emotional upsets, divorce, a higher risk of alcoholism, and other evidences of stress.

But these can be constructive as well as dangerous ages, and the second language of sex has a good deal to offer you if you want to move in new directions in your personal life. Shared tenderness, warmth, humor, merriment, anger, passion, sorrow, camaraderie, fear—feelings of every conceivable sort can flow back and forth in a sexual relationship that has matured to this level of development.

Part of the secret of learning the second language lies in learning how to give. Receiving is much easier. It makes few demands. But the habit of only taking deadens the impulse to reciprocate. As Erich Fromm wrote in *The Art of Loving* (1956), "Most people see the problem of love primarily as that of being loved, rather than that of loving, of one's capacity to love." Giving is *not* an endless gift of yourself to others in which you expect nothing in return. Nor is it a marketplace transaction, trading with the expectation of an equal exchange. Healthy giving involves not only the hopeful and human anticipation that something equally good will be returned but also the pleasures inherent in giving, regardless of the return. The balance to be struck must be chosen by each person and worked out in partnership.

The second language implies sensitivity. It means clearing up long-held grudges and old irritations toward your partner and people in general so that your energy is not wasted in negativity. It suggests the possibility of renewing love every day. It requires knowing what pleases your partner and what pleases you. It involves playfulness as well as passion, and talking, laughing, teasing, sharing secrets, reminiscing, telling jokes, making plans, confessing fears and uncertainties, crying— all in the privacy of shared companionship. In fact, it need not involve the sex act at all.

If boredom creeps into the relationship, both you and your partner need to acknowledge it; it is time to look for or listen to the deeper feelings that each of you has hidden away against the time when the richness of such feelings will be welcome and restorative. You have to *resist* the pulls of habit. Routines and responsibilities may have dulled the impulse to really talk; fight against succumbing to the temptation to withdraw into your own self-absorbed world. Self-centeredness, wanting sexual and emotional contact only when you are in the mood, without concern for your partner's needs, is guaranteed to produce conflict. Competitiveness based on some fancied level of sexual performance is also deadly.

The second language of sex can be developed by actively trying to learn it. Older people may have struggled throughout their lives to overcome obstacles, earn a living, raise a family, and carry out other responsibilities. In doing so they have literally sacrificed their private lives and individual growth to this process. But fortunately love and sex are *always* there, waiting to be rediscovered, enhanced, or even appreciated for the very first time, whether you are young or very old. Self-starters have the advantage over those who wait passively for love to strike like lightning.

Older people have, in fact, a special ability to bring love and sex to new levels of development because they are more experienced. Many people do learn from experience. They develop perceptions that are connected with the unique sense of having lived a long time and having struggled to come to terms with life as a cycle from birth to death. A number of these qualities are beautifully suited to the flourishing of the second language. An appreciation of the preciousness of life and the valuing of immediateness can occur as people become older. What counts now is the present moment, where once it was the casually expected future. If developing an awareness of the brevity of life leads you to come to terms with your own mortality in a mature and healthy way, by no longer denying it, you will find you no longer live heedlessly, as though you had all the time in the world. The challenge of living as richly as possible in the time you have left can be exhilarating, not depressing.

Elementality—the enjoyment of the elemental things of life—may develop in late life precisely because older people are more keenly aware that life is short. Such people may find themselves becoming more adept in separating out the important from the trivial. They might uncover a heightened responsiveness to nature, human warmth, children, music, and beauty in any form. Healthy late life is frequently a time for greater enjoyment of all the senses—colors, sights, sounds, smells, touch—and less involvement with the transient drives for achievement, possessions, and power.

Older people have time for love. Although they have fewer years left to live than the young and middle-aged, if they are in reasonably good health they can often spend more time on social and sexual relationships than any other age group. It is true that many have limited financial resources, but fortunately social and personal relationships are among the pleasures in life that can be free of charge.

Willingness to change counts, as well. It is possible to become quite different in later life from what you were in youth. Obviously, the change can go in positive or negative directions. But the point to remember is that *change is possible.* You do not need to become locked into any particular mode of behavior at any time of life. Experimentation and learning are possible all through-out your life, and this holds true for both sex and love. Naturally, the more actively you grow, the greater the reservoir of experience and the larger the repertoire you can draw upon in getting along with and loving other people.

The early and middle years set the stage, but per-haps only in the later years can life, with its various choices and possibilities, have the chance to shape itself into something approximating a human work of art. And perhaps only in later life, when your personality reaches its final stages of development, can lovemaking and sex achieve the fullest possible growth. Sex does not merely *exist* in the later years; it can become greater than it ever was.

The special psychology of sex in the second half of life will eventually be better understood than it is now. Then we will comprehend for the first time the full life cycle of love and sexuality—with youth a time for excit-ing exploration and self-discovery; middle age, for gain-ing skill, confidence, and discrimination; and old age, for bringing the experience of a lifetime and the unique perspectives of the final years of life to the art of loving one another. We have a great deal yet to learn from those who personally have mastered this complex and wonderful art over years of time.

GLOSSARY

Androgen Any of the *steroid*★ hormones produced by the adrenal glands and the *testes* that develop and maintain masculine characteristics; *testosterone* is the best known.

Anus The opening from the lower bowel (colon) through which solid waste is passed.

Atrophy A wasting away or diminution in size of a cell, tissue, organ, part, or body.

Bartholin's glands Two small, roundish bodies, one on either side of the vaginal opening. Although they produce mucus in sexual excitement, they are not

★Words italicized are defined elsewhere in the Glossary.

the primary source of vaginal lubrication during intercourse.

Benign prostatic hypertrophy (BPH) Noncancerous enlargement of the *prostate* gland that occurs in the middle and later years.

Bladder The distendable elastic sac that serves as a receptacle and place of storage for the urine.

Cervix The part of the *uterus,* sometimes called the neck, which protrudes into the *vagina.*

Circumcision Surgical removal of the foreskin, a loose fold of skin that surrounds the head of the *penis.*

Climacteric See **Menopause.**

Climax See **Orgasm.**

Clitoris A small, erectile organ at the upper end of the *vulva,* homologous with the *penis,* and a significant focus of sexual excitement and *orgasm* in the woman.

Coitus Copulation, coition, sexual intercourse.

Cowper's glands A pair of small glands lying alongside and discharging into the male *urethra.* They contribute lubrication during sexual activity.

Cystitis Inflammation of the urinary bladder.

Dyspareunia The occurrence of pain in the sexual act, usually experienced in the female vaginal area.

Ejaculation The forceful emission of the seminal fluid at *orgasm.*

Ejaculatory impotence Inability to ejaculate.

Erogenous zones Sensitive areas of the body, such as

the mouth, lips, buttocks, breasts, and genital areas, which are important in sexual arousal.

Estrogen One of the active female hormones produced by the *ovaries* and the adrenal glands, which has a profound effect on the generative organs and breasts.

Fallopian tube The tube that leads from each *ovary* into the *uterus*; after *ovulation* the ovum travels through the tube on its way to the *uterus* and fertilization takes place in the tube.

Flashes (or flushes), hot A symptom associated with the hormonal changes during *menopause*, caused by a sudden rapid dilation of blood vessels.

Foreplay Sexual acts which precede intercourse, during which the partners stimulate each other by kissing, touching, and caressing.

Frigidity An imprecise term applied to various aspects of female sexual inadequacy: (1) popularly, abnormal lack of desire, of coldness; (2) inability to achieve an *orgasm* through intercourse; (3) inability to achieve *orgasm* by any means; (4) any other level of sexual response considered unsatisfactory by the woman or her partner.

Genital area The area which contains the external genital organs such as the *vulva* in the female and the *penis* in the male.

Genitalia The reproductive organs, especially the external organs.

Hormones Chemical substances produced in the

ductless (endocrine) glands of the body and discharged directly into the bloodstream. They have specific effects upon the activity of a certain organ or organs. Sexual hormones regulate the entire reproductive cycle. (The body produces many nonsexual hormones as well.)

Hormone therapy The medical use of supplementary hormones (other than or in addition to those produced by the endocrine glands) for treatment of diseases and deficiencies.

Impotence Lack of erectile power in the male *penis,* which prevents copulation.

Labia Two rounded folds of tissue that form the outer boundaries of the external genitals in the female.

Libido Sexual desire.

Mastectomy Surgical removal of a breast.

Masturbation Stimulation of the sex organs, usually to *orgasm,* through manual or mechanical means.

Medical specialties regarding sex:

Endocrinology The functions and diseases of the ductless (endocrine) glands.

Gynecology The diseases, reproductive functions, organs, and endocrinology of females.

Urology The functions, organs, and diseases of the urinary system in males and females and of the reproductive system in males.

Menopause The time of life for the human female, usually between the ages of forty-five and fifty-five, which is marked by the cessation of *menstruation* and *ovulation.* It may be gradual or sudden, and it can last from three months to three years, or even longer. It marks the end of the childbearing potential.

Menstruation   The periodic discharge of the body fluid (menses) from the *uterus* through the *vagina*, occurring normally once a month.

Nocturnal emission   *Ejaculation* of *semen* at night while asleep; often called a wet dream.

Oral-genital sex   Forms of stimulation of the *genitalia* by the mouth:

Cunnilingus   Stimulation of the *vulva* (especially the *clitoris* and *labia*) by the partner's mouth and tongue.

Fellatio   Stimulation of the *penis* by the partner's mouth and tongue.

Orchidectomy (orchiectomy)   Removal of one or both *testes*; castration.

Orgasm   The culmination of the sex act. There is a feeling of sudden, intense pleasure accompanied by an abrupt increase in pulse rate and blood pressure. Involuntary spasms of pelvic muscles cause relief of sexual tension with vaginal contractions in the female and *ejaculation* by the male. It lasts up to ten seconds.

Ovaries   The two major reproductive glands of the female, in which the ova (eggs) are formed and *estrogen,* or female hormones, are produced.

Ovulation   The process in which a mature egg is discharged by an *ovary* for possible fertilization.

Papanicolaou test or Papanicolaou smear (Pap test)   A simple test to determine the presence of cancer of the *uterus* by analyzing cells taken from the *cervix* or *vagina*.

Penis   The male organ of sexual intercourse.

Perineum   (1) The internal portion of the body in the pelvis occupied by urogenital passages and the rectum; (2) the internal and external region between the *scrotum* and *anus* in the man, and the *vulva* and *anus* in the woman.

Pituitary gland   An endocrine gland consisting of three lobes, located at the base of the brain. The body's master gland, it controls the other endocrine glands and influences growth, metabolism, and maturation.

Potency   Sexual capacity for intercourse; the ability to achieve and sustain erection. Applied only to the male.

Premature ejaculation   Almost instant *ejaculation* (within three seconds) upon entry of the *penis* into the *vagina*.

Prostate   A walnut-sized body, partly muscular and partly glandular, which surrounds the base of the urethra in the male. It secretes a milky fluid which is discharged into the *urethra* at the time of emission of *semen*.

Prostatectomy   Surgical removal of part or all of the *prostate*. There are three types, depending upon the anatomical approach: (1) transurethral (TUR); (2) suprapubic (or retropubic); and (3) perineal.

Prostatism, prostatitis Inflammation or congestion in the *prostate.*

Refractory period See **Sexual response cycle.**

Replacement therapy See **Hormone therapy.**

Scrotum The sac containing the *testes.*

Semen The whitish fluid containing sperm, which is discharged in *ejaculation.*

Sensuality The wider aspect of *sexuality;* the involvement of all the physical senses that enhance and express one's sexuality.

Sex (1) Urge for and (2) act of sexual union.

Sexual dysfunction A general term for different varieties and degrees of unsatisfying sexual response and performance.

Sexual fantasies Vivid and excitatory imaginings about sex; healthy and common in both sexes.

Sexual hormones See **Hormones.**

Sexual response cycle The physical changes that occur in the body during sexual excitement and *orgasm.* It includes four phases: (1) the excitement or erotic-arousal phase during *foreplay*; (2) the intromission or plateau phase; (3) the orgasmic or climax phase; and (4) the resolution or recovery phase. The time required for the completion of recovery—the time required before the first phase can be successfully initiated again—is called the *refractory period.* The *refractory period* is more critical to the male.

Sexuality   The emotional and physical responsiveness to sexual stimuli. Also, one's sexual identity, role, and perception; one's femininity; one's masculinity.

Sperm   Spermatozoa, the male reproductive cells, produced by the *testes* and discharged during intercourse into the *vagina.*

Sterility   The incapacity to reproduce sexually; infertility.

Steroids   A class of chemical substances that includes the *sex hormones.*

Testes (testicles)   The two male reproductive glands, located in the cavity of the *scrotum,* the source of spermatozoa and the androgens.

Testosterone   A male hormone (an *androgen*), a *steroid,* produced by the testes.

Thyroid gland   The gland partially surrounding the windpipe (trachea) in the neck whose function is to supply *hormones* that adjust the metabolism of the body.

Urethra   The passage or canal in the *penis* through which the male discharges both urine and *sperm.* In women the passage through which urine passes.

Urethritis   Inflammation of the *urethra.*

Urogenital system   The organs that serve the functions of urination, sexual activity, and procreation.

Uterus (womb)   The hollow muscular organ in the

female in which the embryo and fetus develop to maturity.

Vagina   The tube or sheath leading from the *uterus* to the *vulva* at the exterior of the body. It receives the *penis* during intercourse.

Vaginitis   Inflammation of the *vagina*.

Vas deferens   The duct from each *testicle* that carries *sperm* to the *penis*.

Venereal disease   Any disease that is transmitted during sexual intercourse.

Virility   Masculine vigor, including *potency* (from which it must be distinguished), sexual prowess (skill), sexual frequency, and attractiveness.

Vulva   The external female genitalia, including the *labia, clitoris,* and the outer *vagina*.

Womb   See **Uterus.**

BIBLIOGRAPHY

Allers, Christopher: "AIDS and the Older Adult." *The Gerontologist.* 30(3), 1990, pp. 405–407.

Almvig, Chris. *The Invisible Minority: Aging and Lesbianism.* Utica, NY: Institute of Gerontology, 1982.

———. *For Yourself: The Fulfillment of Female Sexuality.* Garden City, NY: Doubleday, 1976.

Berger, Raymond M. *Gay and Gray: The Older Homosexual Man.* Urbana: University of Illinois Press, 1982.

Brecher, Edward M., and the Editors of Consumer Reports Books. *Love, Sex and Aging.* Boston: Little, Brown, 1984.

Comfort, Alex. *The Joy of Sex.* New York: Crown, 1972.

————, ed. *Sexual Consequences of Disability.* Philadelphia: Stickley, 1978.

Doress, Paula, and Diana Siegal. (Boston Women's Health Collective) *Ourselves, Growing Older.* New York: Simon and Schuster, 1987.

Fromm, Erich. *The Art of Loving.* New York: HarperCollins (Harper & Row), 1956.

Gambert, Steven. "Sex and Type 2 Diabetes." *Medical Aspects of Human Sexuality* 24, May 1990, pp. 20–27.

Gay, Peter, *The Bourgeois Experience: Victoria to Freud.* Vol. 1, *Education of the Senses.* New York: Oxford University Press, 1984.

Goldstein, Irwin, and Larry Rothstein. *The Potent Male: Facts, Fiction, Future.* Los Angeles: Body Press-Perigee, 1990.

Greenwald, Morgan. "The SAGE Model for Serving Older Lesbians and Gay Men," in *Homosexuality and Social Work.* New York: Haworth Press, 1984, pp. 53–61.

Greenwood, Sadja. *Menopause Naturally: Preparing for the Second Half of Life.* Volcano, CA: Volcano Press, 1988.

Hammond, Doris B. *My Parents Never Had Sex: Myths and Facts of Sexual Aging.* Buffalo, NY: Prometheus Books, 1988.

Heiman, Julia, and Joseph LoPiccolo. *Becoming Orgasmic: A Sexual Growth Program for Women.* Englewood Cliffs, NJ: Prentice-Hall, 1988.

Isensee, Rick. *Love Between Men: Enhancing Intimacy and Keeping Your Relationship Alive.* Englewood Cliffs, NJ: Prentice Hall.

Kaplan, Helen Singer. *Disorders of Sexual Desire and Other New Concepts and Techniques in Sex Therapy.* New York: Bruner/Mazel, 1979.

————. *The Evaluation of Sexual Disorder: Psychological and Medical Aspects.* New York: Bruner/Mazel, 1983.

————. *The New Sex Therapy: Active Treatment of Sexual Dysfunctions.* New York: Bruner/Mazel, 1974.

————. *PE: How to Overcome Premature Ejaculation.* New York: Bruner/Mazel, 1989.

Kelly, James J. "The Aging Male Homosexual: Myth and Reality," in M. Levine, ed., *Sociology of Male Homosexuality.* New York: Basic Books, 1979, pp. 253–262.

Kievman, Beverly, and Susie Blackman. *For Better or Worse: A Couple's Guide to Dealing with Chronic Illness.* Chicago: Contemporary Books, 1990.

Kinsey, Alfred C., Wardell Pomeroy, and Clyde E. Martin. *Sexual Behavior in the Human Male.* Philadelphia: W. B. Saunders, 1948.

Kinsey, Alfred C., Wardell Pomeroy, Clyde E. Martin, and Paul M. Gebhard. *Sexual Behavior in the Human Female.* Philadelphia: W. B. Saunders, 1955.

Lark, Susan. *The Menopause Self-Help Book.* Berkeley, CA: Celestial Arts, 1990.

Leiblum, Sandra, and Raymond Rosen, eds. *Principles and Practice of Sex Therapy: Update for the 1990s.* New York: Guilford, 1989.

Levin, Rhoda. *Heartmates: A Survival Guide for the Cardiac Spouse.* New York: Prentice-Hall, 1987.

Masters, William H., and Virginia E. Johnson. *Human Sexual Response.* Boston: Little, Brown, 1966.

————. *Human Sexual Inadequacy.* Boston: Little, Brown, 1970.

Masters, William, Virginia Johnson, and R. Kolodny. *Masters and Johnson on Sex and Human Loving.* Boston: Little, Brown, 1986.

Money, John. *Gay, Straight, and In Between.* New York: Oxford University Press, 1988.

Napier, Augustus. *The Fragile Bond: In Search of an Equal, Intimate, and Enduring Marriage.* New York: HarperCollins, 1988.

National Institutes of Health. *Impotence: Consensus Development Conference Statement.* Bethesda, Maryland, December 7–9, 1992.

Norwinski, Joseph. *A Lifelong Love Affair: Keep Sexual Desire Alive in Your Relationship.* New York: Dodd, Mead, 1988.

Papadoupoulos, Chris. *Sexual Aspects of Cardiovascular Disease.* New York: Praeger, 1990.

Reinisch, June. *The Kinsey Institute New Report on Sex: What You Must Know to Be Sexually Literate.* New York: St. Martin's Press, 1990.

Riley, Mathilda White, Marcia G. Ory, and Diane Zablotsky, eds. *AIDS in an Aging Society: What We Need to Know*. New York: Springer, 1989.

Rosenthal, Saul. *Sex Over 40*. Los Angeles: Tarcher, 1987.

Rothman, Ellen. *Hands and Hearts: A History of Courtship in America*. New York: Basic Books, 1984.

Scheingold, Lee, and Nathaniel Wagner. *Sound Sex and the Aging Heart: Sex in the Mid and Later Years with Special Reference to Cardiac Problems*. New York: Human Sciences, 1974.

Schover, Leslie. *Prime Time: Sexual Health for Men Over Fifty*. New York: Holt, Rinehart & Winston, 1984.

————. *Sexuality and Cancer: For the Woman Who Has Cancer and Her Partner,* and *Sexuality and Cancer: For the Man Who Has Cancer and His Partner,* American Cancer Society, 1988.

———— and Soreu Jensen. *Sexuality and Chronic Illness: A Comprehensive Approach*. New York: Guilford, 1988.

Sherfey, Mary J. *The Nature and Evolution of Female Sexuality*. New York: World, 1973.

Starr, Bernard D., and Marcella B. Weiner. *The Starr-Weiner Report on Sex and Sexuality in the Mature Years*. Briarcliff Manor, NY: Stein and Day, 1981.

Utian, Wolf, and Ruth Jacobowitz. *Managing Your Menopause*. New York: Prentice-Hall, 1990.

Wake, William. Considering the Special Issues of Older Lesbians and Gay Men. Unpublished paper, 1988. Available from author: Send a SASE to William

Wake, BSN, P.O. Box 1782, Old Chelsea Station, New York, NY 10011.

Weg, Ruth B., ed. *Sexuality in the Later Years.* Orlando, FL: Academic Press, 1983.

Whitehead, E. Douglas. "Diabetes-Related Impotence and Its Treatment in the Middle-Aged to Elderly." *Geriatrics,* Part I: 42(6) (1987): 63–73; Part II: 42(7) (1987): 77–85.

Wilson, June. *Eating Well When You Can't Eat the Way You Used To.* New York: Workman, 1987.

Zilbergeld, Bernard. *Male Sexuality: A Guide to Sexual Fulfillment.* Boston: Little, Brown, 1978.

The only medical journal that covers clinical and psychosocial components of sexuality and family life is *Medical Aspects of Human Sexuality.* Although it ceased publication in 1992, it is still a useful reference and can be found in libraries.

A practical, authoritative newsletter directed to the sexual concerns of the mature adult is *Sex Over Forty,* P.O. Box 1600, Chapel Hill, NC 27515.

INDEX

ABOUT THE AUTHORS

ROBERT N. BUTLER

Dr. Robert N. Butler, a Pulitzer Prize winner, has been Brookdale Professor and chairman of the Department of Geriatrics and Adult Development of Mount Sinai Medical Center in New York City since 1982.

As chairman of the first Department of Geriatrics in an American medical school, Dr. Butler is a national leader in improving the quality of life for older people. He came to Mount Sinai from the National Institutes of Health, where he created the National Institute on Aging in 1976 and served as its first director. Under his leadership, the need for federal funding for research in gerontology gained recognition. One of his achievements was the establishment of research programs for the study of Alzheimer's disease.

A prolific writer, he won the Pulitzer Prize in 1976 for his book *Why Survive? Being Old in America.* He is a member of the Institute of Medicine of the National Academy of Sciences, is a founding Fellow of the American Geriatrics Society, and has served as a consultant to the United States Senate Special Committee on Aging, the National Institute of Mental Health, Commonwealth Fund, and numerous other organizations. He is editor-in-chief of the journal *Geriatrics.*

MYRNA I. LEWIS

Myrna I. Lewis is a psychotherapist, social worker, and gerontologist with a special interest in the social and health issues of midlife and older women. She is an assistant professor at the Mount Sinai School of Medicine in New York City

(Department of Community Medicine). She has a part-time private psychotherapy practice in which she specializes in working with men who are presidents of their own companies or chief executive officers. She is also currently a doctoral candidate in social work at Columbia University.

Ms. Lewis writes a monthly psychology column entitled "Feelings," for *New Choices Magazine* for the age group fifty to seventy. She has co-authored with Dr. Robert Butler and Dr. Trey Sunderland, *Aging and Mental Health: Positive Psychosocial and Biomedical Approaches* and, with Dr. Robert Butler, *Midlife Love Life,* as well as a number of professional and popular articles. She makes regular appearances on radio and TV on the subjects of aging and on women's issues and is a frequent lecturer to professional and public groups.